Exhale

Exhale

HOPE, HEALING, and a
LIFE IN TRANSPLANT

DAVID WEILL, MD

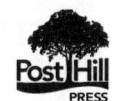

A POST HILL PRESS BOOK

ISBN: 978-1-64293-760-2
ISBN (eBook): 978-1-64293-761-9

Exhale:
Hope, Healing, and a Life in Transplant
© 2021 by David Weill, MD
All Rights Reserved

Cover art by David Gee

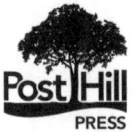

Post Hill Press, LLC
New York • Nashville
posthillpress.com

Published in the United States of America
1 2 3 4 5 6 7 8 9 10

To my daughters, Ava and Hannah, and my wife, Jackie—three people I want most to be proud of me.

To my mother, Kathy, who taught me about the magic of books, a special gift she has given me that is only surpassed by her unconditional love.

And finally, to my father, Hans, who inspired me to believe in myself no matter the circumstance, and to stand up for what I thought was right. All the time. No matter what.

Author's Note

On many occasions, after seeing something at work that is inspiring or upsetting, it has occurred to me what a unique position I've been in, to be simultaneously so close to both the devastation of death and the wonder of what modern medicine can provide. In the pages that follow, I have tried to give readers a window into that dichotomous experience, to give sight to the daily miracles in our midst.

But here's my bottom line, for those that like to read the ending of a book first: Transplant is a miracle but is, at its essence, a human endeavor, performed by people with strengths and weaknesses, powerful attributes and profound flaws. And I am one of those people.

Patients come to see us expecting consistency and predictability. They expect that we will save their lives. But the doctors, surgeons, and nurses doing transplant work have bad days, bad months, and, unfortunately, even bad years. We have fights with our spouses that put us in surly moods and clashes with our colleagues that often have less to do with patient care than they do with power and ego. We get pissed about being cut off in traffic on the way to work, or show up exhausted after staying up all night with one of our sick children. We are just like everyone else, no better and probably no worse. My mistake, at times, was to believe it when patients would tell me that I was "brilliant," "a miracle worker," and even worse, "a god."

We carry around the stresses of everyday life but also the immense burden of being responsible for saving people's lives, of being the steward of the waiting list that determines who will get the next precious organ that—often through a tragedy—becomes available. When things went well, the job didn't seem like much of a burden. In fact, it wasn't like having a "real" job—one where you can't wait until the weekend, or where you always feel underappreciated. Mostly, I couldn't even believe I got paid to do it.

But even when the travails of everyday life interrupt our focus or dampen our moods, we remain responsible for our patients' lives. We bear this burden on good days and on bad days, sometimes elegantly and other times, as you shall see, less so.

Each successful transplant brings a wave of euphoria that surges through our bodies, uplifting our spirits and reminding us why we got into this business. But when things go badly—and things do, even in good transplant programs—it's like having a boulder strapped to our backs and being tossed into a bottomless ocean. At least, that's how it was for me. On those days, they couldn't pay me enough to do it, nor did it comfort me when someone compared me to a deity.

However, through it all, the magic of doing this kind of work for a living is that it means you're giving patients a second chance at life. Helping the courageous patient group I treated was a humbling privilege, and I fought hard to fulfill my duty to them. Showing up for work every day, I made a de facto vow to all my patients: I promised them *air*.

As you read my story, you'll see that this promise wasn't always easy to honor. But doing so has been my life's work and my most important, imperfect mission.

These pages primarily focus on the ten-year period during which I led the lung transplant program at Stanford University Medical Center. But even before coming to Stanford, when I did transplant work at other hospitals, I saw my colleagues and myself at our best and our worst, both brilliant and imperfect. This book is my story, one I've waited years to tell. It is my opportunity to share my experiences, in my own words, from my own perspective.

Just a few ground rules. The events and people I describe to you in the book are portrayed the way I experienced them. With some exceptions, I've changed the names, identities, and other specifics of individuals in order to protect their privacy and integrity, and especially to protect the patients I encountered over the years. The conversations I recreate come from my clear recollections of them, though they should not be taken as word-for-word recitations. Instead, I've retold them in a way that evokes the feeling and meaning of what was said, in keeping with the true essence, mood, and spirit of the exchanges.

I stand behind the truth of what is depicted. Nonetheless, each one of us has his or her own version of the truth. This is mine.

—David Weill
New Orleans

In no relationship is the physician more often derelict than in his duty to himself.
—William Osler, M.D., interview at Baylor University Medical Center

We are all fixing what is broken. It is the task of a lifetime.
—Abraham Verghese, M.D., *Cutting for Stone*

Contents

PART TWO

PART THREE

PART ONE

*Lucky is the man who does not secretly believe
that every possibility is open to him.*
—Walker Percy, *The Last Gentleman*

Prologue

"I am writing to let you know that I'll be leaving Stanford effective July 1."

Send. No, not yet.

I studied the email again, reading and rereading what I had written in the middle of the previous night.

Sitting in my office at Stanford University on a bright Northern California morning, the sun was all the way up, and I would have given anything to be outside enjoying the beautiful morning. Maybe hiking in the Santa Cruz Mountains or riding my bike up the Pacific Coast Highway. But instead I was stuck inside, trying desperately to get an email out of my outbox.

I needed to pause for a moment, to decide for sure that this was what I wanted to do after all these years, all this effort, all the careful crafting of my career. I looked around at the photos on my desk—of my father and mother on their wedding day, my wife Jackie when we were first dating, and the baptism of my younger daughter, Ava. I looked at the poem my older daughter, Hannah, had written in Kindergarten about what it meant to have me as her dad.

I turned back to the computer screen, framed by the brilliant blue sky outside the window behind my desk. *I will miss looking outside at the beauty that surrounded me on this campus, but not what surrounded me every day inside this building.* I took a slow sip from my stainless steel travel mug, inhaling the deep, sweet aroma of coffee and chicory.

"My decision to leave was difficult. I think our team has accomplished a great deal in the ten plus years I have been here. During my decade as Medical Director of the Lung Transplant program, I partnered with many of you to turn around a struggling program and increased the volume of transplants performed while achieving excellent outcomes."

Teamwork sprinkled in with self-congratulations. Excellent. I rubbed my eyes that were dry and red from too little sleep and too much screen time. *Okay, send it.*

Not yet. I can't. I want the words to be exactly right. Only one chance to get it the way I want it—to communicate my message to the people I worked with, both those who were in my corner and those who weren't.

"By their very nature, decisions of this sort are multifaceted and are never about one single thing."

No, this decision is about many things: frustration, burnout, disillusionment. All passenger emotions—the unwelcome byproducts of leading one of the largest transplant programs in the country. For a bit longer than I should have. Longer than those close to me wanted me to.

I glanced at a picture of my family on the front step of our house, Jackie laughing at the camera, Ava in my lap, my arm tightly around Hannah.

Back to the screen. *Focus, David.*

"I am proud of what we accomplished together and hope from the deepest part of my heart that the important work that we do here will continue successfully. Everyone needs a new challenge from time to time, and I am very excited to enter this new phase of my life and to the experiences that lie ahead for my family and me."

Was I excited? Mostly I am excited to get the hell out of here. It has been my crowning professional achievement, true enough. But the price was too high, the physical and emotional debt too costly. It was time for the pilot to eject himself.

But if I'm honest, I have no idea what lies ahead for me.

I read it again from the top. It struck the right tone—not snarky, not apologetic, but gracious, forward-looking. An optimistic turn of the face to a new dawn and toward the warmth of the sun.

Okay, send it then.

Not yet.

"Thank you for your hard work over the years. Our efforts at providing excellence on behalf of the very sick people who count on us have always been paramount. Nothing should get in the way of this vital mission."

Nothing should get in the way, but plenty did. Sometimes other people got in the way—sometimes I got in the way of myself, tripping over my own flaws.

Send.

The ground below came up fast to meet me, and my only thought right then was, *Will the parachute open?*

One

I am a physician, but probably not in the way you envision. I'm not the one performing operations in a surgical gown, like a character out of the television show *Grey's Anatomy*. But there is a lot more to the transplant process. I had a large say in who got the transplant and when, and my team and I cared for the patients from the time they were placed on our waiting list, including managing their post-surgical recovery and then overseeing the care for the rest of the patients' lives. And the responsibility for the administrative duties and the leader of a team comprised of different disciplines and personalities? That was me.

When I met people in the community—whether at my kids' soccer games or at a Palo Alto dinner party—they would ask me what it was like to do my job. Even when I was in the thick of things, I thought a great deal about how best to answer that question. I first gave them the simple answer: that I brought the patients to our program and talked to them about the risks and benefits of getting a transplant; I put them on the waiting list and then selected a pair of lungs for them when a donor became available. But I also said being the head of a transplant program was like being a choreographer, making sure all the dance moves were right. Or like being the play caller—headset on, laminated sheet in hand, prepared for every possible situation. On other days, I would say, it was like being an air traffic controller: coffee in hand, monitoring the planes in the air, trying to bring them all in safely for a landing.

My patients and I have a lifelong bond—a relationship that could be called codependent but was in reality mutually beneficial. They trusted me with their life, to get a new set of lungs and to get them home in one piece—and in the process gave me the education of a lifetime and a heap of gratitude, which will fuel me for the rest of my life. I promised them air, and in return they gave my life purpose, a well-defined mission that never left me wondering if what I chose as my life's work mattered.

When I was a kid and dreamed of being a doctor, I didn't dream of learning anatomy, or doing research, hunched over a laboratory table in sterile isolation. Or even, say, of becoming a pediatrician, which I pictured as seeing one kid after another with a virus of some sort. I wasn't even particularly interested in the premed courses that I needed to take in college in order to get into medical school.

My main motivation was to be a hero, to save the day, to be loved. I know what you're thinking. *He must not have been hugged enough as a child.* No, that wasn't it. I got plenty of love from both my parents, a doctor and a nurse. But I was like the budding actor in film school who wants to be a movie star instead of learning the nuances of acting, studying the great ones, and listening to countless discussions of an actor's method. As a child, I remember my mother telling me that, in biblical terms, the name David meant "Beloved One." I liked that. A lot.

When I decided to pursue medicine, I weighed the pros and cons of all the specialties and all the possible factors, like the length of the residency and the earning potential. But I kept on coming back to one question: *Would I matter?*

The specialty I chose never left any doubt. It was a field in which we were changing the course of a disease, snatching back a life, or—as one of my early colleagues said—pushing back the hand of Jesus. I was relentless most of the time in my pursuit of this discipline, and it worked for my patients and for me.

Until it didn't.

Transplant medicine did more than give me what I wanted and what I needed. It became the vehicle by which I could express myself.

This happened over the course of moments just like this.

Winter 2006
Palo Alto, California

The quiet of the morning, just before the nurses change shifts. The day nurses haven't come in yet, and the night nurses are too exhausted to move or speak. Patients' families are asleep in the waiting room. Except for me, the older doctors—the ones out of their residency—aren't there yet. The only sound that registers, barely, is the rhythmic sound of the mechanical ventilator delivering breath to the new lungs, interrupted only by the occasional sound of a monitor alarm in the distance.

I'm sitting in a chair by a patient's bedside, a young woman named Cindy with cystic fibrosis who received a double lung transplant several hours ago. Just days earlier, near her end, she had been dying a suffocating death, trying to breathe while coughing up cups full of infected sputum. The call about the organ donor had woken me in the middle of the night, just like so many times before. It meant that Cindy could come off the waiting list. She went to the operating room, and then after the procedure was wheeled back to the ICU where I was waiting for her. She is now moving slightly, trying to clear the sedative and anesthetic medications from her system. The lungs are working perfectly, just as I had hoped when I accepted them for her the night before.

Alone with a patient, without the background chatter from the staff, this was always my favorite time in the hospital, or maybe, I should just say, my favorite time—period.

The nurse asks me if I can watch the patient while she grabs a cup of coffee in the break room. I say, "Sure." But inside I'm screaming, *Go, leave me alone—this is the best part!*

The nurse makes a beeline out of the room. My eyes follow her, just to make sure she's gone.

Now it gets better.

Cindy is waking up, eyes searching the ceiling, shaking her head slowly, coughing a silent cough around the endotracheal tube. I stand up and lean over her in the bed, coming into her field of vision from out of nowhere, it must seem. I smile at her, and her eyes sparkle. I tell her that we'll get the tube out soon, that the transplant was a success. That she's a rock star. That I'm so proud of her. Her eyes start to fill with tears. Mine do, too.

I can't possibly imagine a better feeling, a rush you can't get from any pharmacy, or off the street from a dealer, or at a local bar. No, this is different.

And I thought, in that moment: *I could do this again and again—watch a patient wake up from a successful transplant—over and over, and no one would ever tell me to stop.*

Two

Like most good things in life, becoming a transplant doctor happened by accident, without any grand plan or strategic calculation. I took a turn, and suddenly it was there—my new love. And like most loves, you know from the beginning how fragile it is, and sometimes you love so much, so hard, you even expect to lose it one day.

I fell in love with transplant in 1990. It was clear, yellow piss that did it.

Let me tell you the story.

Once upon a time, I was just a kid. Well, not exactly a kid. I was twenty-six years old, a month removed from my medical school graduation and three hours into my internship at Parkland Memorial Hospital in Dallas. (Yes—*that* Parkland Hospital, where President Kennedy had died.) The program director gathered us fresh interns together and told us that, because one of the fifth-year residents had become seriously ill, he needed one of us to volunteer to staff the kidney transplant service. My hand shot up instantly, and I was "hired."

Talk about getting too far over your skis—I hadn't even figured out where the johns were yet, much less being anywhere near equipped to manage a kidney recipient.

Nonetheless, the hubris of youth led me to the assignment that would change my life. Off I went.

Then I thought about it for a moment.

This is insane. I didn't know much medicine, but I did know that transplant medicine is not the bunny slope. Given the complicated physiology involved when transplanting an organ from one person into someone else, and the added complexity of immunosuppressive drugs, there was no way I could contribute anything meaningful to these patients' care; in fact, I thought I might be at risk of harming them. However, having been conditioned to take on challenges by my father and my medical training, I accepted.

"Got it, Chief. Ready to go. Tell me where to."

"Report to Dr. McGinnis in Nephrology. Lots of patients to see. They're talking about doing a transplant tonight." As fate would have it, our team *was* planning to do a kidney transplant that night, my very first night on call.

"Where is the kidney uni—?" My question trailed off as our residency chief walked away. "No problem, Chief, I'll figure it out," I said to no one in particular. "And don't worry, I'll do a hell of a job." *Thank God the hospital has great malpractice insurance for us interns put in undoable situations,* I thought. I hoped I wouldn't kill anyone that night.

Before reporting to my new assignment, I walked to my call room to pick up my backpack. The dormitory-style room smelled of unwashed residents and was littered with unread medical journals and discarded, soiled scrubs. There was a single bed and a small desk, both of which struck me as funny during my residency: a bed in which I would never be able to sleep, and a desk at which I'd never read. In those days, young doctors didn't learn at a desk or on a computer. They learned at the patient's bedside.

I found the kidney transplant unit ten minutes later. Ryan McGinnis was there, talking with Bobby, the middle-aged man who was going to receive a transplant that night. He was emaciated; his limbs were like four sticks poking out of the hospital gown.

Just as I walked up, I heard him say, "You mean afterwards…there'll be no dialysis?"

"That's right. If all goes well," Dr. McGinnis replied. He was too busy writing in the chart to catch Bobby's reaction, which was a combination of disbelief and excitement. Realizing how much his life would change, I became excited, too.

"No dialysis, ever?" Bobby leaned in closer, speaking louder this time.

Dr. McGinnis looked up and stared at him blankly for a few seconds. "No, not if everything goes according to our expectations."

"Well, Doc, let's make sure everything goes right, okay? And who's this?" he asked, pointing at me.

I was standing behind and to the side of Dr. McGinnis, who turned around. Before he could say anything, I stepped forward, extended my right hand.

"I'm Dr. Weill. I'm the intern on the kidney transplant service." We shook hands. Dr. McGinnis looked me up and down, probably wondering how an intern got assigned to his service instead of a more experienced resident. "I'll be helping take care of you tonight. Everything is going to go fine. Excited?"

"You bet I am, but I'm not sure about an intern taking care of me."

Dr. McGinnis stepped forward. "Don't worry," he reassured him, "I'll be supervising him, making sure you're all taken care of. Any questions?"

Bobby shook his head no and looked at me, still not quite sure.

I put my hand on his arm just as the transporters came to wheel him from the waiting area back to surgery. "I'll see you a little later, okay?"

Bobby looked at me and said nothing. Dr. McGinnis walked away from the bed, and I followed closely.

I hustled to the residents' library and found a relatively recent book about kidney transplant. Leafing through it, I tried to absorb as much information about postoperative care as I could. I was interrupted by my pager going off every few minutes, but I learned a few principles. The first priority post-surgery was to get the patient peeing. New kidneys: have to make sure they work. To hasten this process, the protocol was to give the recipient enough fluids for him to urinate, but not so much as to drown his lungs. I didn't know exactly how much that would be, but I guessed I'd figure it out.

For the next few hours, I took care of other patients while waiting for Bobby to get out of surgery, addressing fevers and changes in mental status and admitting new patients to the hospital. When one of the nurses called to let me know that he had come through successfully, I ran up eight flights of stairs two steps at a time to the kidney transplant unit. I couldn't wait to see if this man would pee, but I was terrified about the very real possibility that I would make a mistake. My pulse was racing, and I thought my heart was going to beat out of my chest. In spite of my inexperience, I was going to be in charge of a new transplant recipient for the next eight hours.

I got to the kidney unit just as Bobby was being wheeled back, the surgical team at his side. After telling the nurses a few details about the operation, the surgical team left. As one of the younger surgeons passed me, he smiled and said, "Call me if you need me, need me if you call me, but remember: calling me is sign of weakness." I laughed nervously. This was something of a hospital mantra at Parkland that I would hear, and say, hundreds of times in my three years there.

I strategically placed my chair right in front of the bag that would collect Bobby's urine, and for the next few hours I just sat there, periodically getting up to talk to the nurses who were trying as hard as I was to stay awake. While waiting for this guy to urinate, I was afraid to go to the bathroom myself, concerned that I might miss something, so I just sat there.

When Bobby woke up from the anesthesia, I asked him repeatedly if he was in any pain. He kept his eyes closed and mouthed the word "no" each time I asked. So as not to bother him any further, I decided to go down to the cafeteria on the first floor to get some coffee, happy to stretch my legs.

When I got back twenty minutes later, I drank my coffee slowly at the patient's bedside, staring at the urine bag. Before I reached the bottom of my Styrofoam cup, it happened—urine happened! I jerked forward in my seat. I never thought I would be so excited to see yellow liquid passing into a Foley catheter bag—slow drips at first, and then a steady stream. I turned my back to see if anyone else was seeing what I was, and then turned back to the bag. It was filling up and beginning to bulge out. I lifted the bag and squeezed it, feeling its warmth with my hand, and smiled.

Turning to the nurse twenty feet away, I said, "Hey, this guy is making urine! Unbelievable!"

She didn't look up from her paperwork, just took a long sip from her coffee and said, "Great. I'll notify the newspapers. And keep it down—the other patients are sleeping."

But who could sleep? I was amazed. Transplants actually *worked*. I decided to wake the patient to let him in on the big news.

"Bobby, can you hear me?" I shook his shoulder. "Guess what? Your kidney is working. You're starting to make urine."

This got his attention. He opened one eye. "Huh?" he said, still groggy.

I told him again.

This time he opened both eyes and said, "I haven't made urine in a long time. Don't joke with me."

"I'm not. It's true." I rushed to empty out the urine bag into a plastic container and showed it to him. "See?" I said.

"Well, I'll be damned." I grabbed his shoulder, and we both smiled.

That night, both our lives changed. An indigent patient from South Dallas on Medicaid would be going back to peeing naturally, no longer requiring dialysis three times a week. And I, a young intern from the suburbs, had just experienced the magic of transplant—the way it could transform a patient's life in an instant, from sick as hell one day and on the road to recovery the next. I saw that it was more than just the replacing of a body part—it was the giving of a new way of life, with unlimited possibilities. Isn't that what all doctors sought when they decided to go into medicine?

And so it happened. A jolt of transplant "lighting" had gone right through me, and I was hooked. Giving the gift of hope that night, playing that small part in Bobby's care, sparked a flame that would burn hot in me for the rest of my career.

What would I learn after that night in Dallas thirty years ago?

A lot.

As my career unfolded, I didn't see transplantation only from a doctor's perspective—one that would have allowed me to keep some cold, clinical distance. I saw it in my own family when my father received a liver transplant in 2001. At the time he received his transplant, he was a professor of medicine at a large academic institution, had the medical knowledge to research anything he wanted, and had a transplant doctor for a son. And yet he knew very little about what was going to happen to him and what eventually did happen.

How does one get a transplant? How does it *really* work?

Well, as I've seen in my experience taking care of transplant patients in some of the country's best hospitals and now in my consulting work helping transplant centers improve, it's complicated.

To really understand, patients need to appreciate the complex nature of transplantation and consider all the influences that various stakeholders have on the process. As we say in my home state of Louisiana: It's quite a gumbo.

First, you need to know the players: the groups that impact the transplant patient as she goes through the process. There's the large, multidisciplinary transplant team of doctors, nurses, social workers, dieticians, physical therapists, pharmacists, and other healthcare personnel. And, as with any large group, everyone brings their own set of unique talents to their job each day but also their ego, insecurities, and biases.

There are the hospital administrators who run the hospital. Most with whom I have interacted are good people, but they are running a business—sometimes quite a big business—so they are balancing patient care with business decisions.

Then there are the insurance companies. These are businesses as well. I've talked to a lot of these folks, too. They generally aren't bad people either, but they have to answer to their own boards of directors and, in many cases, Wall Street.

Finally, there are the government regulators. Transplantation may be the most heavily regulated field in medicine, and transplant programs must satisfy certain requirements to stay in business. So, when the regulators say, "Jump," the transplant programs usually say, "How high?" I'll talk about how this impacts patient care.

At the center of all these forces is the patient, who just wants to survive.

Don't misunderstand my message. These influences can come together and get the job done, aligning their interests for the good of the patient. But when the various interests become misaligned, it creates a situation that is not good for patient care—and, frankly, isn't pretty to watch.

This narrative leads you through the transplant process—and it is a process—as I have done with thousands of patients over my career. But for the attention-challenged among us, here are the basic steps: One, have a disease that is amenable to transplant. Two, get a physician to refer you to a transplant center. Three, get evaluated by a transplant center (and you'll need good health insurance to reach this step, let alone any beyond it). Four, get on the center's waiting list. Five, get a call about a donor picked out especially for you. Six—and this is the big one—get a transplant operation. Seven, survive the surgery and beyond. Simple, right?

Just as I shepherd transplant patients and their support network of family and friends through this process, this book shares what I saw, what I was thinking and feeling while I saw it, what my patients experienced, and what I learned. Most days on the job I thought, *I wish everyone could see what I'm seeing.*

And how was it to do this job? To help people get a transplant successfully?

The best job in the world.

But at times devastating.

I can say this: I never once had trouble getting out of bed to go to work, never once had to think about how to make my job more interesting, more meaningful. Sure, there were days and nights that I can only classify as an ass-whipping, when I was so tired that my prevailing thought process was: *bed, coffee, bed, coffee.*

I saw some great things happen, even helped make some great things happen. I discovered wonderful things about myself and others. And some horrible stuff. I'll remember both for the rest of my life. It was the education of a lifetime.

Would I do it all again? Yes, without hesitation, qualification, or conditions. But, first, maybe some ice cream and Netflix, followed by a nap.

But before I go any further, you might want to know a little bit about me, and then I'll get to the cool transplant stuff.

Three

Growing up, I knew my father liked that I played sports. Basketball was a way to earn his approval—something I craved; it was a way for me to know my father was proud of me and, in some ways, to gain his respect.

I went with my father to most of the New Orleans Jazz home games. The Jazz was our local NBA team, but in essence it was shooting guard "Pistol Pete" Maravich surrounded by a bunch of guys. We would cheer on our team, despite their perennial losing record, yell at the refs, share popcorn. In the '70s, it was okay to give a kid a sip of beer, and my father would laugh at the silly face I made after I took too big of a swig.

My father admired the good players. He wasn't much of an athlete, hobbled by congenital hip deformities that would eventually require four hip replacements. Most of his experience with sports came from watching other people play, including me, and he came to my high school games when work didn't get in the way. I always knew when he was there—and noticed when he wasn't—although he didn't yell and scream from the sidelines as some parents did but would just give a slight smile when I made a good play. My mother was a different story. She would yell at the refs when they made a bad call against me. She didn't like anyone messing with me—then or now.

During my senior year of high school, we beat our archrival, and I scored the winning basket. I looked up in the stands as our bench and our fans went bananas and saw my father, a taciturn German Jew, give me a quick fist pump—for him, the equivalent of a backflip.

School was my father's thing, or more precisely, being smart was his thing. I wasn't much of a student, which would have made my father proud, given how much he valued his own intellect and his own academic success. I wasn't interested in studying in high school and didn't become so until college, when I had nothing else I could use as a way to get his attention.

He was a quintessential Old World intellectual: loved books, classical music, and philosophy. Some of my earliest childhood memories are of him in his office at home, listening to Mozart, sitting quietly at his desk, either reading or writing in longhand on a legal pad. His mind was agile, precise, and disciplined. And he could use it for good or to criticize someone or something that wasn't up to par. I was on the receiving end of both.

The most obvious place where he used his mind was in his profession. He was a lung doctor, just like I turned out to be, but he was a different kind—a scientist, a researcher who rarely saw patients. I think sick people, with all the many ways they can manifest and react to their disease, were too messy for him. They rarely followed a pattern or a predictable course he could control. My father became a star in his field, an occupational lung disease researcher who traveled the world to lecture and received all the accolades associated with this sort of career—an extensive publication record, recognition in his specialty, and large research grants. His success was quite obvious to me, even when I was young. I was acutely aware that my first male role model set the bar high.

The comfort I experienced growing up in an upper-middle-class suburb of New Orleans was the opposite of the uncertainty he faced as a young boy. Raised in wartime Germany, my father got an early close look at what humans were capable of doing to one another. I think it hardened him, resulting in him muting his emotions to protect himself from feeling hurt again. I believe the horror of watching his father being taken away to Buchenwald, the details of which he insisted remain unspoken throughout his life—despite my innocent probing—shaped his thinking. These child-hood experiences made him feel "other." I, on the other hand, lived the ultimate high school boy dream—good at sports, popular, and unencumbered by doubt or fear of failure.

My mother's early life experience was quite the opposite of my father's. She learned to value the heart, human experiences, and emotions, and cared deeply about other people. Her compassion may have been a reflection of growing up in Selma, Alabama, the small town that would eventually become a symbol of the civil rights movement. She wouldn't walk by a person of color, or anybody else for that matter, without asking them how their day was going, making them visible when I am sure, at times, they felt invisible.

And she was smart, an avid reader of books on all kinds of topics, which sharpened her practical mind and ordered her world—and our family's—in a most empathetic way. She would start reading when we left for school each morning, saying goodbye to my sisters and me from a chair, with her legs up on a footstool, her cup of coffee within reach. My mother enjoyed the silence of reading, and she later told me she used books all her life as an escape, particularly when she was a girl growing up with an alcoholic father who could be abusive when drunk. She read to grow and to learn, to feed her mind and her heart. I remember that, even as a child, I would often hope that I had my father's brain but my mother's heart.

As I completed high school, my dreams of playing basketball in college began to fade. The kids playing college ball were not only bigger, faster, and stronger, they were also just better. After my senior-year basketball season ended, my focus shifted to debauchery. My group of friends and I found all the bars in New Orleans were willing to serve alcohol to seventeen-year-olds, and we frequented them as often as possible. I fit the stereotype of a typical high school jock, chasing cheerleaders (and non-cheerleaders, for that matter) and carousing on the weekends. New Orleans was perfectly suited to these kinds of adventures. But as graduation approached, I reluctantly started to consider my future.

I hadn't put much thought into picking a college. Most of my peers were going to prestigious schools in the Northeast, or at least reputable universities in the South. They'd done their homework, reading all the brochures and diligently touring college campuses. In contrast, I had only visited the University of Florida in Gainesville. There were two reasons for that visit: I could stop in Destin, Florida, on the way, where my family had a condominium near the beach, and the school had a good football team. My best friend David joined me, which was not particularly memorable except for the tour of the football stadium and getting a flat tire on the way back. Ultimately, I didn't even end up applying there.

In the end, I applied to Louisiana State University (LSU) in Baton Rouge, Tulane University in New Orleans, and Trinity University in San Antonio (where my oldest sister, Judy, was in her fourth year). I was accepted to all three: LSU because, at the time, all Louisiana residents were accepted; Tulane because my father was on the medical school faculty; and Trinity for reasons that still aren't clear. I decided on Trinity because my sister was there, and San Antonio was known for excellent Mexican food.

I remember the night before I left for college, I walked through the living room and saw my dad smoking a Cuban cigar on the patio—his post-dinner ritual. The Cuban embargo didn't stop him; he smuggled them in via a Swiss tobacconist he met in the '60s while lecturing in Zurich. Growing up, I would sometimes watch him out the window from our upstairs kitchen and wonder what he was thinking. Most nights, he sat perfectly still for a half hour, methodically putting his hand to his mouth and puffing away, slowly smoking the cigar all the way down. This was his time to think alone, away from the family. He was a man who needed his space. The thick smoke that surrounded him on that patio every night seemed symbolic of how hard it was for me to feel close to him. To this day, the smell of cigars brings me back to our home in New Orleans, to that patio.

This particular night, he spotted me through the French doors that led from our living room to the backyard and summoned me to his poolside "office."

"Have a seat," he said.

Oh shit, I thought. Whenever my father spoke like that, I was in for an uncomfortable conversation. When my father had something to say there was no wind-up, usually just fast balls—high and tight.

"Okay," I said. "What's happening?" I sat down tentatively.

"I want to talk to you about college."

"Yeah, I'm ready to go. Got all my stuff packed. Looking forward to it. Should be fun." I guided the conversation to the logistical and the operational—a conversational smoke screen. It didn't work.

He waved his cigar at me as if to tell me to shut up. "I want to talk about the academic part." Smoke swirled up from his lit cigar, burning my nose. He took another draw. "You haven't exactly been a great student, not because you can't do it, but because you lack discipline. That's got to stop." He blew out the smoke right over my head, nearly choking me. "You can't just continue to fuck off and expect to do anything with your life. Do you even know what you want to study?"

"I was thinking about premed," I answered. I had worked in a local hospital as an orderly over the summers and observed the doctors, some of whom were my father's friends, and thought to myself, *That looks cool. These guys are studs.* But that night was the first time I had said out loud that I wanted to be a doctor, and as soon as the words left my mouth, they immediately sounded ridiculous. I could have more plausibly said I wanted to play quarterback for the New Orleans Saints or lead a space expedition to Jupiter.

My father didn't let me get away with the silliness of the comment. "Yeah, premed. Right." He took a long draw, raised his eyebrows, rocked his head back, and rolled his eyes mockingly.

I had thought he might be pleased to hear this—most fathers would kill for their sons to be interested in what they do. He wasn't, though, because it seemed like wishful thinking. Nothing I'd done in school so far had shown I could do the hard work that medical school required.

"I'm only going to say this once: When you get to college, you better get it together. Get in the library every night—ass in chair. Quit all the fucking off, the bars, whatever the hell it is you do. If you don't, you'll be nothing. You'll be working in a shopping mall." He leaned back, finished. Message delivered.

I sat there thinking about what he had said for a minute, wondering if I had it in me to study the way he wanted me to and imagining what it would be like to work in a mall. There would probably be a food court, I figured, so maybe it wouldn't be all that bad.

I tried to refocus but couldn't think of anything to say.

"Okay, Dad," I finally managed. "Good night."

I walked back to the house, still mulling over what he had said. He had given me a challenge. No way was I going to back down.

Off to college I went, for a year at Trinity, and then, missing home, I returned to New Orleans to finish my bachelor's degree at Tulane. My college experience was unexciting but pivotal. There was not much in the way of partying or college girls. I had turned into a grind—a straight-A student who burned to excel in my newfound academic game. I had traded the basketball court for the classroom—same drive, different sport.

I graduated a semester early from Tulane. I was in a hurry to finish college, taking courses all summer long, wanting to get to the next step of applying to medical school. I applied and was accepted to a number of schools, but only one was of any interest to me: Tulane. It was a good medical school and, most importantly, tuition-free for me, since my father was on the faculty there. At that point, I was just grateful to be going to medical school anywhere.

Four

"D r. Weill, will you come up and read this chest X-ray for us?"

I was a first-year medical student sitting in the back row of an auditorium filled with my classmates and several faculty members who were occupying the front rows. The faculty, called "attendings" in the academic world, were fully trained in their specialties. From my vantage point in those early days in medical school, they were gods—all-knowing and full of confidence and wisdom.

We were learning that day about chest X-rays—the basics: how they were shot, what one could see on them, and which parts of the radiograph correlated to what body part. It was essentially X-rays 101.

When I heard the professor call out, "Dr. Weill," I stayed planted in my seat, peering over the other students so I could see my father get up and show the class how to read the chest X-ray. He was in the first row, with the heads of departments—whom I considered real studs—talking with the professor leading the class. I couldn't hear what they said, but both were smiling and nodding.

"Dr. Weill, please come up and read this X-ray." All the deities in the front turned around and looked at me. Then all my classmates turned and looked at me, too. *What are they looking at?* I thought. It dawned on me after a few beats. *Wait—Fuck! They expect me to come up and read the X-ray! They can't be serious.*

My closest medical school friend, Del Dressel, was sitting next to me. He elbowed me and said, "I think they mean you." He started to laugh, and soon the others around us joined in. I stood up, my heart racing, my legs heavy, and made my way to the front of the auditorium. On my way up, one of the smartest people in the class—a woman from Southern California, whom I considered an egomaniac, said sarcastically, "Go read the X-ray, *Doctor* Weill." The "Doctor" part of how she addressed me seemed preposterous at the time—I knew as much about being a doctor at that point as the guy cleaning the laboratories at night.

I took my place in front of the light box used to read X-rays. The light from the box was heating the skin on my face to what felt like a thousand degrees. Having to perform for this room full of real and future doctors was like trying to interpret a chest X-ray on the surface of the sun. Sweat formed on my lower back. I half-turned to look over at my father, who smiled slightly, nodded, and tilted his head toward the light box.

Turning my attention back to the X-ray, I started to speak, feeling a hundred pairs of eyes on me, all boring into the back of my head. Suddenly, I recalled a memory that might just help me get through this. When I was a kid, maybe ten years old, I would join my father on his Saturday morning rounds at Charity Hospital. He would bring a group of pulmonary trainees to the radiology department, a dank space in the basement, where they would review

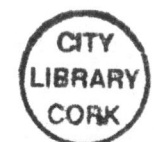

patients' X-rays. My father gently criticized the young doctors when they screwed up, but mostly in good humor. He would stand next to the trainees reading the film, pointing out findings—as well as cajoling them when necessary. I only once saw him really go after one of his trainees, berating him in front of the whole group for a mistaken interpretation. I don't think it was the misinterpretation that set him off but the lack of interest—the trainee's seeming not to care. Lack of effort and lack of commitment—these were two of my father's least-favorite traits.

Here I was now, a trainee myself, reflecting on those childhood days more than a decade ago when, instead of running around and climbing trees with other kids, I had spent time examining X-rays in a dark room with my father and his minions.

I started to speak, remembering to call out each physical structure and to be systematic and organized as I interpreted the film, just like my father had directed those young doctors back then. Starting from the outside and working in, I said softly, "The soft tissue and bony structure look good"—without knowing whether they actually did, I at least knew to start there. No one stopped me, so I continued. "The trachea and mediastinum look good." Still no interruption, so I kept going. "The heart looks…" *Let's see*, I thought. Then I recalled my father, spinning around on a stool in the X-ray room, saying that the cardiac silhouette—the shadow the heart makes on a chest X-ray—is a normal size if it's less than one-third the width of the entire film. "The cardiac silhouette is…maybe…a bit enlarged." I heard nothing, except a sort of grunt from my father in the first row. *Hmmm, I* thought. *I must be getting this wrong.*

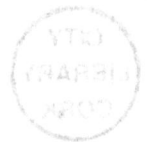

I continued: now to the lungs, which I had no clue how to interpret. "The right lung is normal," I said with surprising—and unfounded—confidence. Then loudly, "And the left lung is normal," as though I possessed some sort of metaphysical certitude. I turned around to face the front row, to indicate that I was done.

The professor walked over and looked at the X-ray, and then at me.

"*Doctor* Weill, why don't you look at the left lung again?" I turned again to the lightbox, convinced that I had missed something—maybe even something obvious. I scanned the left lung but couldn't see whatever I had missed the first time. It was like asking me to read Mandarin. Honestly, I might have had a better chance with Mandarin.

I turned and looked at the professor pleadingly. I raised the white flag. He paused for a few moments, leaving me to dangle. He used his pointer to circle a quarter-sized abnormality in the left lung, obscured slightly by the cardiac shadow, which, I would later learn, is a classic way a chest X-ray can mask a cancer.

"A lung cancer, Doctor," stated the professor. "Congratulations. You just missed a potentially curable cancer in your patient." The entire auditorium laughed, and I looked over at my father, who was smiling.

"You can sit down now," the professor added. I made my way back to my seat and sat next to Del, allowing my heart rate to settle back down.

"Nice job, dickhead." He gave me a push on the forehead. "You just killed that guy." I smiled.

"Probably won't be the last one."

At the end of that day, I went back to my locker to get the stuff I would need to study that night. Inside my locker was a red textbook. *How did that get there?* I wondered. I looked at the front cover. The title was a classic of pulmonary medicine, *Diagnosis of Diseases of the Chest* by Fraser and Pare, which describes how lung disease appears on a chest X-ray. My father had taped his business card to the front of the book, with the simple inscription, "You may want to read this." I looked through the large tome for a few moments, feeling its weight and flipping through one radiographic image after the next. It was several hundred pages and dense. I left the card where it was and placed the book in my backpack.

I started reading it that night. And would soon read it cover to cover.

That was medical school for me. Long hours in the hospital and library, sure. That's medical school for everyone. But mine included a special kind of scrutiny, being Hans Weill's kid. When a test didn't go well, it was Hans Weill's kid who'd struggled. This may not have been what my professors were thinking, but that's how I looked at it. And when I started to excel, especially during the clinical rotations in my last two years, well, that's what was expected. It was certainly what I expected, but I also always knew it was what my father expected of his only son.

Five

Fall 1995
Denver, Colorado

"It's showtime, motherfucker," a male voice announced as I picked up the phone.

The person greeting me so "warmly" on the phone that night when I'd been asleep was Marty Zamora, a faculty member designated as the lung transplant pulmonologist when Dr. Fred Grover, a cardiothoracic surgeon, came to Denver to start the program.

"We have a good donor—right blood type, right size, right lung function. Right night," Marty explained. I would find out this was "typical Marty." It was early enough in his transplant experience—every doctor in the country's transplant experience, really—to be genuinely excited each time a lung donor offer came through for a patient.

I was fast asleep at 3:00 a.m., only a few hours removed from a night out at the Cruise Room, my favorite bar in downtown Denver. I had been hanging out with my friends, guys with whom I was doing my pulmonary and critical care training at the University of Colorado. The university was recognized as the top place in the world to get training in

33

everything related to the lung—clinical care to cutting-edge research. Since I'd received good recommendations from the attending doctors in Dallas during my residency, I was able to secure a spot in this storied training program. My father, being an internationally known lung doctor, was pleased with this development—not only because I was entering his field, but also because I would be training in Denver. He knew many of the lung doctors and had trained the chief of pulmonary, Dr. Marvin Schwarz.

I started out with the idea that I would pursue my interest in lung transplantation. Fortunately for me, the University of Colorado had recruited Dr. Grover to build the lung transplant program there. It was one of the first in the country, starting a year or so prior to my arrival. I had decided to go to Denver because of its world-class training in pulmonary disease and its new specialty in lung transplantation.

I became the first doctor in the long history of pulmonary training in Denver to dedicate one year of the three-year fellowship to lung transplantation. The preferred route for pulmonary trainees was to develop a laboratory-based research career. However, after a few months in the lab, I was bored out of my skull, and so spent many afternoons riding my bike when I should have been doing rat experiments and collecting data. Since this was a new lung transplant program, no one previously had had an opportunity to dedicate twelve months to learning what was still being discovered at the time about lung transplantation. I floated the idea of spending my last year focusing on lung transplantation to Dr. Schwarz. He was a legend in the pulmonary world, not only for his considerable medical expertise, but also for his sharp (and politically incorrect) humor.

"So you've decided to be a complete scumbag?" he asked. "Yes," I answered. And off I went.

And that excitement spread quickly to me, not just that night at 3:00 a.m., but for many nights to follow. It was like suiting up for the big game, or even more dramatically, for the big battle, especially in those early days when one was never really sure what would transpire on the night of transplant. At times it seemed like the drill was, "Put the lungs in and let's see what happens." The procedure wasn't exactly experimental—it was a bit beyond that. But not much beyond that.

My transplant year in Denver was busy because I was on call every day. To add more difficulty, Marty's wife had developed complications from a brain tumor, and he often needed to take care of her at home. He was always available for questions by phone, but many nights I was on my own to figure things out.

One patient in particular turned out to be a real education in my new specialty. We had done a single lung transplant on a fifty-four-year-old former smoker with emphysema named Catherine. The operation had gone well, and she was recovering without a hitch in the ICU on postoperative day one. I went by to check on her in the late evening before I went home. As I walked into the room, I found her sitting up in bed talking with her husband. "There's my favorite doctor, Doogie Houser." She wasn't the first patient to compare me to the adolescent doctor on the popular TV program of the same name.

I smiled. "Good evening, Mrs. Ellis. You look good tonight."

"Look good, feel good," she responded. Her husband rose to greet me, extending his hand. "You guys did a great job, Doc. Tell the whole team thanks."

I looked at the two of them, beaming in their postoperative glow. They knew, and I knew, that the outcome could have been much different. Only a few days before she had been actively dying, sliding right down the path toward a suffocating death.

"We'll move you out of the ICU tomorrow if all goes well tonight. You done good."

I looked over at her, and we locked eyes.

"Don't know how to thank you," she said.

I walked out of the room thinking, *Wow, this transplant stuff is the bomb. I don't think this will ever get old.*

A few days later, after being transferred out to the transplant floor and doing well, Catherine was back in the ICU. I went by to see her, but this time the circumstances were not so rosy. While out on the transplant floor, she had received an accidental but toxic overdose of an antibiotic, Gentamicin. This class of antibiotic, even when carefully dosed, could be harmful to the kidneys (nephrotoxic), a temporary condition that can easily be reversed by decreasing the dose given or the time interval between doses. In this case she had, due to a nursing error, received five times the usual dose and now would need dialysis. This occurred before so much attention was paid to medical errors in the medical literature and the mainstream media.

Although this happened more than twenty-five years ago, medical mistakes remain common. Medical errors are now the third leading cause of death in the United States, accounting for around 250,000 deaths per year, according to some estimates. I couldn't help but imagine what our country's response would be if that many deaths occurred due to terrorist attacks every year.

In this case, the dialysis would likely be temporary, but Catherine would need to be on it at least two weeks while her kidneys recovered. But she didn't want dialysis. She refused to give consent for it, saying she would rather die than be "hooked up to a machine."

I went to her room to try to talk her into getting the treatment. After explaining to her and her husband that she needed the dialysis to survive—and even going as far as to promise her a full recovery—she still refused. Despite his best efforts, her husband also couldn't convince her to change her mind. I called Marty.

"Tell her she's getting dialysis," Marty barked into the phone.

I explained the situation and how adamant the patient was about no further treatment. I told him she was lucid and understood the consequences of her decision.

"Okay, fine, I'm coming over there." Marty announced.

I waited in the ICU, expecting nothing less than the verbal equivalent of a thunderstorm with massive flooding. I wasn't wrong.

Marty walked by me without a word and went straight into the patient's room. Through the glass door of the ICU room, I could see him addressing the couple, gesturing and talking loudly enough for me to hear him but not loudly enough that I could make out what he was saying. Her nurse had joined them, standing at the bedside across from Marty.

After just a few minutes, Marty and the nurse came out of the room. Both of them were unhappy, but for different reasons.

"We gave her that lung. It's ours. I'm not going to stand by and let her commit suicide," Marty said as he looked for her chart, likely wanting to document the conversation. The nurse listened and then gave her own take.

"She can clearly make her own decisions. She's not impaired, she's…"

"She is impaired. She's suicidal."

"Maybe she's had enough. We can't tell her what to do. It's her choice."

"No, it's not. It's *my* choice."

The nurse looked around to see if anyone else had heard this. The head ICU nurse, Val, an experienced nurse who had seen it all, walked up to us. She tried to get Marty to calm down. I got up from a desk at the nurses' station and stood next to Marty as the four of us figured out what to do next.

The head nurse took a turn. "Marty," she said, in the calmest possible voice, "it would be unethical to continue. This is a patient choice issue." She paused. "Because of the stickiness of the situation, I have called an ethics consult so they can weigh in." I looked over at Marty and actually thought I could see steam coming out of his ears.

"A fucking *ethics* consult? Are you kidding me?" he said with disgust, as though she had asked Charles Manson or Ted Bundy to drop by and consult with us about our patient.

Almost on cue, the head of the ethics committee, Charles Alexander, walked up. A highly respected radiologist, he also was universally liked.

"Marty, David. How's it going?"

I said, "Fine," but Marty didn't even acknowledge him.

"I hear you have a bit of a situation."

"No situation at all, Charles. A patient is trying to kill herself, and I'm not going to let her. It's simple."

Dr. Alexander adjusted his glasses and started slowly, trying to reframe the situation. "Marty, I understand the clinical situation. A patient who received a lung transplant, did well, and then had a nephrotoxic dose of antibiotics. She needs dialysis but refuses." Realizing Marty wasn't going to respond, he turned to me.

"Yep," I said, "that's about it." I merely confirmed the facts, but Marty shot me a look that was along the lines of, "Shut the fuck up."

Now talking only to me, Dr. Alexander said this was a clear case of a patient's right to dictate her care—it was patient choice, clear and obvious. We couldn't put her on dialysis against her wishes.

I thought a second to myself. *She's going to die. The first death in my transplant training. A patient whom I got to know before and after transplant, a family I've grown close to.*

Dr. Alexander continued. "We can bring the case before the entire ethics committee, but this one is cut and dried. It would be unethical to continue."

Marty rocked back on his heels, clearly pissed. "An ethics committee? Give me a break." He looked at the nurses who had gathered, then at Dr. Alexander, and then finally at me. "You know what, *I* am the ethics committee on this service. A committee of one." And with that he stormed out the automatic double doors of the ICU. As he departed, he said to us, "Go ahead and kill her if you want."

We all just looked at each other. No one knew quite what to say. After a few moments—which felt like hours—the nurses went back to their stations and Dr. Alexander came over to me and put his hand on my shoulder.

"Look," he said. "Marty is invested, heavily, in these patients. Perhaps too much. Go in and talk to the patient and tell her we will honor her wishes." I thought for a moment. *If I do that, will Marty choke me to death?* I just nodded, and he left the ICU.

I looked through the glass door into Catherine's room and saw her husband at the bedside holding her hand. I went in and sat down on the edge of her bed. Before I began, I turned to look at her husband, who stood behind me. "You have the right to decide what happens next with you. It's your life, and you get to decide. You probably know we want you to fight on, but if you don't want to, we'll pull back."

She nodded. "Alright," I said as if to convince myself that we were actually going to honor her wish. "We're going to make you as comfortable as possible. We'll make sure you pass away as comfortably as possible. Do you understand?" She looked at me with a blank stare. *Was she fully comprehending what I was saying? Or were the cognitive effects of renal failure beginning to develop?*

I didn't let my mind linger there too long—I could have run out of the room and claimed to the nurses that she wasn't mentally competent to make the decision and we should force her to get dialysis. But I didn't. She knew what she was doing. She was choosing death over life—the antithesis of *her* choice to get a transplant, the antithesis of *our* transplant mission. She had broken the unstated pact we had made.

I said goodbye to Catherine and her husband and left the room. There was no going back.

She died peacefully a few hours later.

My first loss of a transplant patient made me feel like a failure, like I hadn't fulfilled the mission. It didn't feel like someone had made a "choice" that they had the "right" to make. It didn't feel that way at all. It felt like someone had kicked me in the crotch. Hard.

The entire episode raised my awareness of a central tenet of the ethical treatment of sick people: patient autonomy—the right of patients to make decisions about their medical care without their healthcare provider trying to influence the decision.

In the end there were no legal ramifications from the nurse's error that had caused this situation—which is usually the case. If all medical errors were brought into the legal arena, malpractice premiums, health insurance, and hospital charges would certainly go up, increasing the trajectory of the unsustainable path we're already on in terms of healthcare costs. We would also need to build a significant number of new courtrooms.

Our team came close that night to violating not only the legal standard of care, but the ethical standard of autonomy. Our transplant team ultimately allowed Mrs. Ellis to exercise her autonomy—we didn't sedate her and start dialysis against her wishes (which I'm now ashamed to say was contemplated)—but this allowance was not our first instinct. *We're transplant doctors,* we thought, *we gave her the organ.*

It's ours—we determine what happens to it. This is wrong, which I hope goes without saying. It is obvious to me as I look back at an event from over twenty years ago. I can tell you it was less clear in real time. We felt that we owned the organ—the machinery keeping a person alive. In effect, we were saying we owned the patient. *Once you get one of "our" organs, you become ours.*

It was an important lesson for me as a young doctor. It was a one of those life lessons that often arises in the course of doing this unique sort of work, a lesson that should be top of mind for all healthcare providers. I wish I could say this type of attitude—the patriarchal relationship between transplant patient and transplant doctor—is a relic of the past.

But it's not.

My transplant fellowship was marked with a dizzying array of all possible outcomes. There were patients who did well, recovering as though they'd had a simple appendectomy rather than a replacement of their breathing parts. Then there were other patients, those who got the operation, got deathly sick, resulting in a slugfest for weeks in the hospital, as we tried everything in the book to get them better—without even necessarily having a textbook to follow.

There were long nights of lung donor transports: flights over the Colorado mountains in snowstorms, with the plane bouncing all over the sky. I recall throwing up on Dr. Grover's shoes one night—after which he decided to wear his OR shoe covers whenever he flew with me to pick up organs. There was the time I was speeding back to Denver with a set of lungs in the trunk of my car, with the music blaring, having a blast, until I got pulled over for going 110 mph. I got out of the ticket and instead received a police escort to the hospital after I opened the cooler and showed the officer what a fresh pair of lungs looked like up close.

Or the time I called a patient on our waiting list who, after a few calls, I found in a bar in a seedy part of Denver, drunk to the point of near unconsciousness while still strapped to his portable oxygen tank. We agreed that it might be best to wait until another night to perform his transplant. I should have warned him then about the colorful conversation he and my boss would have in clinic the following week. Let's just say Marty was unimpressed by his life choices.

I had an eventful year during which I saw and learned a lot. I was fully trained and felt more prepared than I likely was, but it was time to go out and get my first real job.

As I was leaving my training period, I had to quickly learn more than the medicine. I needed to learn how transplant really worked—how programs are set up; how they fit in the larger hospital administrative, financial, and political environments; and most importantly, how the transplant team is built and, ideally, how it functions together.

Six

How do the disparate parts of a transplant program come together to make the transplantation a success—a miracle in plain view? As I would come to find out, the answer to this question was less about the medicine I had taken so many years to learn and more about team dynamics and the alignment of interests within a given hospital.

The transplant field started as a research endeavor that was primarily based in academic medical centers. The pioneers in the field started by doing transplants in animals. I can't overstate how difficult it was to get transplants done in humans, how courageous the medical teams and patients were to try them, and how far the field had come by the time I entered it. Since I entered the field of lung transplantation in the early 1990s, a relatively early time in its development, I was able to witness much of its evolution.

You need three components to make a transplant program a success: a dedicated medical team, an experienced surgical team, and a committed hospital administration. Sounds easy, right?

It's not.

Very few medical centers around the world are able to put all three components together and *keep* them together for any length of time. To give you an idea of how difficult this is to do, consider that there are around sixty lung transplant programs in the United States, but twenty of them account for 85 percent of the total volume of lung transplants performed in this country. This means a small number of centers drive the field, even though many more centers would like to do lung transplants because of the financial impact they have on a hospital's bottom line and the reputation enhancement that results from having a successful transplant program.

The medical team is where I come in. Over the years a lot of my patients have mistakenly thought that I was their surgeon, because I've been their main point of contact within the program. The surgical team is typically busy with other cases, both transplants and non-transplant related, so like in other specialties, it doesn't have as much interaction with patients as the medical staff.

Our job is simple to describe but difficult to do: evaluate patients who might need a transplant, decide if they should get one, pick suitable donor lungs for them, and—here's the really hard part—keep them alive while on the waiting list and for as long as possible after they get their transplant.

The surgical team members are usually cardiothoracic surgeons who also perform all types of heart surgery, scheduled cases involving complex heart repairs, which sometimes divert their attention from their transplant duties. They need to be specifically trained in lung transplantation and to have performed a significant number of transplants under the guidance of a more experienced surgeon. This training is usually done during an extra year, after the resident has completed their usual training in cardiothoracic surgery and focuses entirely on learning not just the surgical technique, but also how to judge organ donor quality and the likelihood that a potential recipient will do well after a transplant.

To be clear, some surgeons do transplants without the dedicated training in the transplant arena, instead learning transplant as part of their cardiothoracic training experience. Depending on the skill level of the surgeon, this may be fine, but there are certainly examples where the surgical expertise is not what it should be. This is true in all walks of life: people are performing jobs where the training for the job has been suboptimal. Except that in the transplant field, the skill levels of the practitioners matter more than they do in most jobs—akin to airline pilots, who can kill hundreds of people if their skills are not up to par.

Regardless, in modern transplant programs, the surgical role is more finite than in the past, primarily centered around the transplant surgery itself and less around the pre- or postoperative care of the patients that can hopefully last many years. I don't want to diminish the role of the surgery. Quite to the contrary. In a transplant program, if the surgical team doesn't do its job well, not much else matters.

I've been fortunate to work with some great hospital administrators during my career, and, not surprisingly, some not-so-great ones. Their role is to first identify transplantation as a hospital priority and then adequately fund it. It's expensive to run a transplant program. The cost is mostly related to personnel: doctors, nurses, nurse practitioners, pharmacists, social workers, dieticians, and program administrators, and depending on the size of the program, there can be a lot of them. Many transplant programs that fail are underfunded, resulting in not enough staff to care for the number of patients being treated.

Even if a hospital has all three of these components, that does not necessarily mean that the program will be a success. There's a final, surprisingly difficult step: getting all three teams to work together. One would think this should be fairly easy, since all should be motivated by the simple goal of getting a patient transplanted successfully. In many instances, a lot can get in the way of this objective: jealousies, egos, personality clashes, loss of focus, and key members leaving the program to go on to greener pastures, to name a few.

Transplantation is a complicated dance, in which the choreography is key. My role as director of the program is to be the choreographer.

Seven

I watched her chest rise and fall, a twenty-five-year old woman named Kim with cystic fibrosis, slowly bringing air in and then letting it out. Rhythmic, mesmerizing, wondrous. I stared for a while longer.

I was the medical director of a new lung transplant program in a large private hospital in North Dallas called Medical City. Hired by a group of cardiothoracic surgeons straight out of my training in Denver, I was young, at thirty-two, to understand let alone take on that level of responsibility. When they offered me the position, I accepted, considering only briefly whether I was up to the task.

Everything started out great. When our program first got going, in the same year that I started, we did very well. We were attracting patients to our center, and we quickly became the most popular transplant program in Texas. My colleagues and I enjoyed working together, and some of us became close friends outside the hospital. After spending the previous ten years struggling as a trainee in the university setting, I began to enjoy the comforts of working in a private hospital. They paid me good money and gave me a lot of autonomy, especially for a young physician just out of training.

I watched from Kim's bedside, becoming a bit self-conscious, feeling like a voyeur—some kind of lung stalker. I would occasionally look over at the nurse, her back to the patient, alternating between fiddling with the drips or inputting data into the bedside computer.

She was missing the show, I thought. I recalled what my father had told me when I was a little boy, putting his stethoscope on my chest: *You breathe in, you breathe out. Simple, right? Amazing, right?* He would let me listen to the sound of my own breathing. A smile would come across my face, and then a giggle. I would ask him if we could keep doing it, and he said, "Sure."

Then I would listen to my father's chest. He would take a few breaths and then hold one in to see if I would notice. When I would look at him, confused, he would shrug and look at me as if to say, "What's the problem?" I would then hold my breath until I couldn't anymore, and then I'd gasp for air, laughing while also trying to catch my breath. "Breathing," he said. "So simple, unless you can't." The smile would leave both my face and his, and I'd think about that for a moment. And start to worry. *Who can't breathe? Doesn't everyone have to breathe?* I reminded myself to think about this some more.

The transplant patient in the ICU directly in front of me was just several hours post-op. She was breathing on her own now, the ventilator disconnected, the tube removed from her throat.

I had seen her the previous night right before her transplant. She was scared, crying, breathing shallow and fast. I held her hand and told her to slow down, that help was on the way. Two new lungs were being flown in, "especially for her—a perfect match." Her parents were with her, and I reassured them. "We got this," I told them. I think I even said it would be "a walk in the park," as if it were a sure thing. We would put a dying patient under anesthesia, take her diseased lungs out, and put in two new/used lungs we pulled out of an ice chest that we had flown in from a hospital a three-hour plane ride away.

This interaction had been just hours ago, and I watched her breathe now in the calm of the moment, the morning sunlight streaming through the ICU windows. I reminded myself, *Never use the phrase "a walk in the park" again.*

I was only hours removed from that morning's victory lap in the ICU. Kim had been pulled from certain death by our team, and her parents were hugging me and telling me I had saved their daughter's life, that I was a miracle worker. I had believed them. Now, at the end of a long day, I was explaining to Jackie, my girlfriend and future wife, why I wasn't in the mood for a night out or anything other than the prone position.

Earlier that afternoon, our team had performed a second transplant in less than twenty-four hours. This time it was on a man in his mid-fifties, Curtis, whose transplanted lungs weren't working at all. He had developed a complication called primary graft failure that results in the lungs basically flooding soon after the transplant. It was a fairly common complication, but one for which we had no explanation. But when it did happen, look out.

For me it meant hours at the bedside, caring for a patient who would likely die, trying anything to save them, including extracorporeal membrane oxygenation (ECMO). This is a mechanical circuit that pulls the blood out of a person, oxygenates it, and then sends it back into the body. ECMO is effective temporarily, but it's certainly not a long-term solution. It is more like a Band-Aid—albeit a nasty, expensive, and risky one, essentially leaving you waiting for various supportive therapies, or divine intervention, to kick in.

"I get it. Remember, I'm a nurse." Jackie looked at me, exasperated.

Suppressing my tendency toward sarcasm, I said, "No, I didn't forget that. But thanks for reminding me anyway."

"You can't crawl under a rock every time one of your patients gets sick."

That got me going again. I spit the words out. "He's. Not. Sick. He doesn't have a sore throat. He's on fucking ECMO."

"Fine. You stay here and wallow in it. I'm going out." She grabbed her coat, and I heard the door slam. I wasn't mad at her for leaving, nor was I surprised. In fact, I was mostly jealous. She was off to live her life. I was staying in to mourn impending death. A few minutes after she left, I got up and went back to the hospital. It was time to go on death watch.

Twelve hours later, after our team had tried every trick we had to save him, I put Curtis back on the transplant waiting list, to see if we could get him a new set of lungs, which was the equivalent of hitting the reset button.

But we couldn't get a set of lungs in time, and he died.

I came back to the apartment and had breakfast with Jackie. We talked about the day ahead, nothing in particular. We avoided talking about my patient. I think Jackie didn't want to appear insensitive to what I was experiencing but still had her life to live, one built out of our shared hopes. She probably worried, even then, at the start of our relationship, that the demands of my job would likely get in the way of a normal life together.

Eight

B rian was one of the first patients I saw in Dallas. He was nineteen, shy, and had an undefined developmental disorder that made him slur his words and seem emotionally immature and unintelligent.

His type of lung disease looked a lot like cystic fibrosis but was actually bronchiectasis, a destruction of the lung airways from multiple infections as a child. His frequent pneumonias were growing harder and harder to treat, and with each infection, his lung tissue was further destroyed.

Though Brian clearly needed a transplant to survive, many other lung transplant programs had evaluated him and were hesitant to put him on their waiting lists. Post-transplant medical care for any organ is complicated, and lung transplants in particular pose unique challenges. Patients must be compliant with the strict regimen, taking medications on a set schedule, being vigilant in avoiding infection, and seeing our team frequently for regular check-ups. Before I arrived in Dallas, the transplant team had concluded that Brian wasn't up to what would be required. They simply didn't think he was smart enough to manage his post-transplant life.

When I came on the scene, I started combing through the records of patients whom we had turned down for transplant and came across Brian's file. He had no medical problems, aside from his obvious lung disease, and was young, with involved parents who took care of him 24/7. After carefully reading his chart, I decided to take a chance on him. Medically, I thought we could successfully perform the transplant. Also, transplanting Brian would show the new team that we wouldn't do things the conventional, conservative way. I pasted a sticky note to his chart that read "Full Evaluation," a signal to the nurses to make an appointment for him to see me. I closed the chart and slapped my hand on the front cover.

Brian came to see me with his parents. When they arrived, his mom waved away my extended hand and went straight for a full embrace. I leaned in a bit awkwardly, giving her a half-hearted hug. While we talked, she held Brian close to her, her arm wrapped around his waist. It was obvious she was familiar with guiding him through stressful situations, and I could tell she loved her son in the way that only someone who had sat up night after night with a sick child can understand.

I had seen this many times with young patients who had been sick all their lives; their illness became a family disease, strengthening the bond between child and parents. My understanding of this dynamic deepened when I had children of my own and could begin to empathize even more strongly with these parents. I would try to imagine what it would be like to hold the hand of my own child drowning in vile phlegm, wondering whether to go to the hospital or ride it out until morning.

Brian's mother was remarried to the best kind of man Texas had to offer—the strong, plainspoken, rugged sort. His handshake firm and enthusiastic. I sat down facing the family and smiled, starting in on the pre-transplant spiel I'd refined through the years.

First, I always tried to get a sense of the patient, to find out if and why they really wanted a transplant. I wanted Brian and his parents to "do well" in this initial consultation, hoping he would be the type of patient I would want to save. Others who were less committed, and frankly, less gutsy, had given up on him. I wanted to be the one to accept him for transplant. But I needed him to prove he could handle taking care of himself after surgery.

"I'm Dr. Weill, Brian. I want to talk with you a bit about getting a lung transplant. I've read your medical records, and it seems you've been sick a lot."

Brian quietly giggled and then looked away, blushing.

"Is transplant something you're interested in?"

He was now bright red.

"Brian, answer the doctor," his mother said.

Brian seemed much younger than his age. I gave him my best nonthreatening look, trying to recall what they had told us on our pediatric rotation in medical school was the best way to get kids to talk. I got closer, put my hand on his shoulder, and dropped the doctor persona.

"So Brian, my man, what do you say we replace these lungs? Get you some new ones?"

"Um, I don't…I guess…Will it hurt?"

"The incision," I said, drawing on my chest with my finger, "will hurt some"—an obvious understatement—"but we have good medicines for the pain, and it won't last long.

We won't let you hurt." I wanted this scared kid to share my confidence, to believe in "us"—even if the only one who was cheering for him on this one was me.

"I don't want it if it's going to hurt," Brian said.

"Sounds reasonable. I'm not here to talk you into getting anything you don't want, but let me ask you a question. Is there anything that you can't do now that you would do if you could breathe better?"

This had become a trademark question of mine over my career. I usually tried to work it into the first few minutes of my conversation with a new patient. It allowed the patient to dream for a minute, to envision a new life, one without the limitations imposed by end-stage disease. The patient's response helped me to understand what he or she truly valued. It was also a great way to get patients to talk.

"I want to run," Brian said as he looked away, seemingly embarrassed.

"Oh, cool. Like run a race?"

"No, just run. I've never done that."

I was still smiling at that point, but this stopped me cold. This kid was nineteen, and he'd never actually run—never chased after another kid or run to the ice cream truck.

I pursed my lips and shook my head. This sucked, and I wasn't going to have it.

"Well, Brian, I think we can help you. If you want to run, let's get you a new engine. Replace the bad breathing parts."

I was now in full swagger. This was for the benefit of the patient and the patient's family, but it also helped me. It was as if I were gearing up for a boxing match, gloves on, mouthpiece in, hitting myself upside my head. Maybe if I said it with enough certainty and determination, it would come true.

"Okay. Mom, is that okay?" Brian asked.

His mom was now smiling, tears running down her face. "Sure, Brian, that's okay with me. Doctor, what's next?"

After giving the mom a more committed hug, the step-dad a firmer handshake, and Brian a fist bump, I left the room and found our nurse coordinator.

"Anne, let's discuss Brian's case at our next selection meeting," I said. "I think we should take him."

"That is so cool, I am so excited," Anne said. "I just love him. The family is so sweet." Anne was in charge of scheduling patients' transplant evaluations, putting them on the waiting list, and doing the myriad other tasks necessary to coordinate the patients' care: scheduling and getting the results of many tests, answering patients' questions, and, most importantly, providing reassurance and interpreting what we doctors said into plain English.

"The first patient you put on the waiting list here, David, couldn't have been a better one," she said.

"Well, not quite yet," I said. "Let's see what everyone says at the selection meeting on Friday. Still need the Good Housekeeping seal of approval."

The main purpose of the Friday meetings was to give the thumbs-up or thumbs-down on a prospective transplant recipient. Disagreements over who should be transplanted were not uncommon and could get heated. These meetings provoked a lot of huffing and puffing by an impressive collection of egos.

This was my first Friday meeting at my new job, but I knew the drill from my training in Colorado—same show, different channel. The team would hear not only about patients' clinical situations, but also about whether and how much they drank, smoked, or did drugs. We would learn whether a candidate was a "good" patient, that is, was compliant with their treatments, had a job, and where and with whom they lived. Patients' characters were a prominent part of our discussions—too prominent, in my opinion, especially given the flaws of the people in the room, myself included. This was our time each week to make life-or-death decisions, all while sipping coffee and devouring mediocre muffins.

I didn't want to take anything for granted. A new hospital, a new team—I had no idea how the selection meeting would go. Nonetheless, I was excited. Beyond just wanting to help this kid, I *needed* to help this kid.

He got to me in a personal way, an occupational reality I would experience many times in my career, and one I would need to learn to manage. It was part of the protective equipment necessary to be safe at the job, like the harness for the window washer on a skyscraper, or protective earplugs for a construction worker who jackhammers all day. But the first step in self-protection is knowing that you need it.

Nine

Two days later, I went to the selection meeting. There were at least thirty people in all—and most stumbled in a few minutes before the 7:00 a.m. start time. Some had been up all night with sick patients or a new transplant.

These meetings, held in a wood-paneled room with a big conference table, were part medicine, part theater, part poker game. Ten chairs around the table were for the more senior physicians, while the additional chairs off to the sides were for the non-physician members of the team, creating a kind of observation gallery for the events taking place.

First patient up for discussion that morning was Brian. I presented the details of his case, shading the presentation—a practice I'd learned long ago to persuade colleagues—as I went. The method involves highlighting the good (his sweetness, his family support) and downplaying the bad (his intellect). He had some "learning challenges," I said, but a "committed family," and he had always been "compliant with his medical regimen." These were buzzwords I knew to use. I was trying to make it so the team couldn't say no.

I thought my presentation was convincing them until I stopped talking and was met with silence. One of the old-guard physicians finally said, "Should we transplant someone who is mentally ret—I mean slow, or whatever he is? Not too many lungs to go around."

I shot him a hard stare. He looked back at me without blinking. "I'm just asking," he said unapologetically.

It was Joseph Peterson, one of our surgeons, a veteran in the cardiothoracic surgery field. The dark hair cropped close to his head contrasted sharply with his incandescent green eyes, which seemed to bore right through me as he talked. He knew the intimidating effect of his stare.

He didn't know it, but this form of intimidation wouldn't work with me. My father had inoculated me against wilting under pressure. I had become a master at techniques of defusing and deflection, but my favorite was humor.

"Well, he is a bit slow, so he would be the perfect cardiothoracic surgeon," I said to a room full of cardiothoracic surgeons, my brand-new colleagues, most of whom I barely knew. "Except I didn't see a lobotomy scar."

Silence around the room. Then, thankfully, one of the other surgeons laughed and most of the others followed. I sighed with relief. I glanced over at Dr. Peterson to see his reaction. He wasn't laughing. *That's okay*, I thought *My first brushback pitch—a fastball intended to spook the batter.*

I went on to advocate strongly for Brian, telling the team it wasn't really our place to make judgments about a patient based on their IQ.

"A life is a life," I said. "Who are we to put a value on it?"

Sadly, we do routinely place values on lives as transplant doctors. We wield the power to choose to save a life or not, and we couldn't save everyone. I've always felt this kind of power should be used judiciously. Back then, this power was one of the few responsibilities in my life that humbled me.

After some logistical conversation among the nurses and social workers about how Brian would know which medicines to take (color code the pill bottles), and how he would get to the clinic each week (Mom and Dad, of course), the rest of the team gave the go-ahead, and we listed him for a transplant.

As we moved on to discuss other patients, I kept thinking about Brian. I couldn't wait to tell him and his parents that he was on the waiting list.

On the way out of the meeting, Anne grabbed my arm tightly, barely able to control herself. "I'm going to call Brian's family right now!" she exclaimed.

"Don't worry, I'll take care of it," I replied.

Anne looked deflated. She loved giving patients the good news. But she understood that I wanted to make this call; she knew that Brian's story had resonated with me and she had seen how hard I'd fought for him. Dr. Peterson, on the other hand, was less elated.

"Well, I guess we'll see," he said to me, tossing his coffee cup in the trash. "I hope it works out."

I reckoned he didn't think it would. To some with whom I've worked, being right is more important than seeing a good patient outcome, even when lives are at stake. It's sad, but true. I sincerely hoped Brian would do well, too, but even today, I can't help but wonder if I cared more about being the hero to his family—about myself—than I did about him.

Much sooner than we expected, just eight days later, the call came. It was midnight, and I was still in my office. A set of lungs were offered to us from Houston, due to a self-in-flicted gunshot wound to the head of a teenage boy. Upon hearing that, I paused for a moment, to think about the pain his family must be experiencing, the yin and yang of trans-plant, someone's tragedy turning into someone else's miracle.

Brian's mother answered my call on the first ring. She started crying before I could get the words out that we had lungs for Brian. Unable to speak, she handed the phone to her husband, who got right down to business. "Got lungs, Doc? Okay, we're coming to the hospital now."

Before I let him hang up, I asked to speak to Brian.

"Hey, hey," I said, "we're going to do the transplant tonight. You ready?"

Brian tried to speak but only stuttered, unable to get words out. I sat on the phone and waited. I remembered reading somewhere that you're not supposed to interrupt anyone if they stutter. Finally, he said softly, "Dr. Weill, I'm scared."

I swallowed hard, tearing up. I was happy that no one was there to see me. *Transplant doctors aren't supposed to cry.* Standing up from my chair, still holding the phone, I looked out my office window and saw a man sweeping the court-yard outside, working the night shift as a hospital janitor. Now *that* was hard work. He saw me looking at him and I waved. He waved back.

"Well, we're not scared, Brian," I said. "The team is pumped and ready to go. We have found you some world-class, Olympic-gold-medal lungs, and they've got your name all over them."

"Really?" he said. He giggled a little.

"Well, no, we don't put your name on the lungs, this would really screw them up, but they're yours."

He laughed, louder this time, and both of us relaxed some.

"See you soon, Brian," I said and hung up. I put the phone down, closed my eyes, and took a deep breath. Brian was going to get a shot at learning how to run.

Ten

While Brian was in surgery, I periodically went to the waiting room to update his parents, telling them that things were going well and he should be out soon. They were grateful for the updates, though they didn't look any less worried after each one. Earlier in my career, I sometimes went into the operating room to see how things were going, but later I would just pace around the hospital, trying to think of possible scenarios that could come up, playing out in my mind how I would react to each one.

After seven hours of surgery, at around 9:00 p.m., Brian came back to the ICU. For the next several hours I stabilized him, making sure the new lungs had the best opportunity to work and that all his other organ systems were not taking a nosedive, as they have a tendency to do after a transplant operation. For most of the night I paced around his bed, looking back and forth between his ventilator and the IV bags hanging above him. At around 2:00 a.m. I pulled up a chair next to Brian's bed and dozed off.

"Doctor, what do you think?" a voice asked.

I opened my eyes to see Louise, Brian's nurse, standing in front of me. I immediately looked at the bedside monitors, hoping I hadn't missed something that had gone wrong all of a sudden.

I took a quick scan of Brian and the bedside monitor. He was stable—his breathing was steady and slow, unlabored. The monitor showed an oxygen saturation level of 95 percent. Excellent. His postoperative course was going better than even I could have hoped. Usually it would take a day or two to get the lungs to work this well after a transplant, but in Brian's case, it was only several hours after his transplant.

"Let's extubate him. Take these new lungs out for a spin."

Louise pushed the call button and told the unit secretary that we needed a respiratory therapist. These hospital personnel, who help out with the ventilator and the extubation process, would take Brian's breathing tube out and disconnect him from the ventilator. We waited on the therapist in silence, both of us looking at the bedside screen that gave a continuous readout of vital signs and oxygenation. I stood up, yawned, and did a deep squat—my ass was killing me from sitting there all night—and then patted Brian on the shoulder.

"Hey Brian, it's Dr. Weill. You awake? No time for sleeping."

His eyes slowly tracked toward mine. They were glassy, but he was in there somewhere. He nodded slowly.

"Are you in pain?" I asked.

He slowly shook his head no.

"What do you say we try your new lungs out?"

Brian nodded yes, this time more enthusiastically. I gave him back one quick, exaggerated nod, the kind I used to reassure patients that everything was under control, a fighter pilot's show of confidence.

Disconnecting a patient from the ventilator always makes me anxious—even now, after all these years—but on this particular day, disconnecting the first lung transplant patient at my Dallas hospital, I experienced sheer terror. Nonetheless, I'd been damned if I was going to show my emotions to either the patient or the nurse.

As Louise prepared for the big event, I went through the automatic double doors to the waiting room and found Brian's parents whispering to each other, alone in the empty room. Seeing me, they both immediately stood up, reading my face for clues about how their son was doing. When I started to smile, the tension dropped from their faces.

"Brian is doing fine," I assured them. "Right on course. In a minute I'm going to try to let him breathe on his own. No guarantee it will work now, but he's in a good position to give it a try."

"Everything's going so fast. Two days ago, he could barely get out of bed, coughing his head off. Now he's got new lungs. It's a miracle," Brian's mother said. *Just doing my job, ma'am.*

Brian's stepdad wanted to know when they could go in and see him.

"Let's wait until the nurses get things tidied up," I said. This was a euphemism for, "Let's make sure he's not gasping for air when we take the tube out and we don't have to scurry around trying to shove the tube back down his throat while we get the ventilator reconnected with you guys standing there."

I smiled. "I'll have someone come get you in just a bit."

When I returned to the ICU, I found a crowd in Brian's room. The respiratory therapist was ready with his extubation equipment and was waiting on me. I stood there for a minute, looking at Brian and the others in the room, then back to the monitor and back to Brian.

"Are you ready, doctor?" Louise asked.

I rocked up on my tiptoes and back again, a habit I'd developed in grade school when I was nervous or thinking hard about something, or both. "Take that sucker out. Let's let this boy breathe." This comment was a show of bravado, but the drama of this first extubation in Dallas was important to me—I wanted to feel and celebrate each moment, to make it memorable.

The respiratory therapist told Brian to cough, and as he did the therapist pulled the tube out. His eyes watered, but he was breathing just fine. He looked around the room, looking a bit self-conscious as we all stared at him. I came right up to him and got my face next to his.

"Brian, you did it. Everything went great. You're a stud."

He smiled, still a bit floppy from the narcotics, and said, "Hey, *we* did it—just like you said."

The drama of these moments, and the satisfaction of seeing a patient's life not only saved but changed forever, made it so I never needed an alarm clock. Each morning, I got ready for work in a dark house, long before the better-adjusted people of the world were awake. But I didn't envy the late sleepers, didn't want to be like them. We were transplanting people's lungs. But can one be too committed to something that is done for a noble purpose: to save someone's life? Can even this kind of pursuit become unhealthy?

I would find the answers to these questions years later.

Eleven

I also evaluated a patient named George for a transplant soon after my arrival in Dallas. George had a disease called scleroderma, which results in one's own antibodies attacking the lungs and several other organs. Because this disease involved many parts of the body, scleroderma was not, especially in the mid-1990s, considered amenable to lung transplant. Even after replacing the lungs, the patient still suffers from the other manifestations of the disease, some of which can be life-threatening.

When George came to see me about a transplant, he arrived with quite an entourage: his mother and father, brothers and sisters, and several aunts and uncles. One of the nurses had to bring extra chairs into the clinic room, and by the time everyone had a place to sit, we couldn't close the door because some of his family were seated out in the hallway.

Before our clinic visit, I had read his medical record. He had already been evaluated by several transplant programs—some local and some on the East Coast. All had reached the same conclusion about his suitability for transplant: thumbs-down. While reading his record closely, I realized his other problems associated with scleroderma really weren't that bad. I thought we could get him through both the operation and the recovery period. I was excited to think we could do something innovative, something on the edge—it was a great way to save a life while we also made a statement about the boldness of our new program. I was young enough and naïve enough to believe we could get it done.

Many objective measures go into determining if someone is a good transplant candidate. The best candidates are those who have only one organ system that isn't working, so when you replace the bad organs, the patient does well. Most of the transplant evaluation is directed at just this—measures of how one's body will stand up to the rigors of a transplant operation and recovery. We test all the organs in various ways, using blood tests, imaging studies, and other objective measures.

The one thing we can't measure that may be equally or more important than the objective criteria is the subjective one: Does the person have the "right stuff?" Can they withstand the rigors of the regimen from a psychological and emotional standpoint? The question becomes: Are they tough enough?

A burgeoning field of transplant medicine concerns the psychosocial evaluation of transplant candidates. This type of evaluation, now supported by a robust body of literature, rightly concludes that patients who have strong family and friend support systems, who do not abuse alcohol or drugs, and who have complied with previous complex medical regimes make better transplant candidates.

That's the easy part. The hard part, which there is no objective way to determine, is how the patient will respond when the transplant is not working well, and they need to hang in there until it does, or when they are in pain, or when they need to stay in the hospital a long time to recover. I try to imagine a patient not doing well when I first meet them. How will they respond? Will they circle the drain when times are tough? Or will they fight like hell with all they've got? I've seen both responses from patients, and the ability to withstand, to dig in, is the difference between living and dying after a transplant. I do this same assessment in my own life: who can I trust to be there when the shit hits the fan, who will really be there and dig in as I confront life's biggest challenges.

I don't know how I assess the inner workings of my patients' minds—I couldn't teach my trainees this skill, although I would have liked to. I could only tell the doctors I mentored that they needed to have this sixth sense to be successful in transplant medicine. I use this sense when I meet people for the first time outside of the hospital setting, without necessarily wanting to, or even being conscious of it. I imagine people with a life-threatening illness or even in wartime. How would they respond? Another example of how my "transplant mindset" has leaked into my civilian life.

Knowing this, I first wanted to meet George, to look him in the eye and see for myself if he was up to the challenge.

I could tell right away, from the first time I met him in our clinic, that he was. He told me that he got out of bed each morning before sunrise, strapped on a backpack containing his oxygen tank, and went off to work in his family's Mexican restaurant. He worked until closing time, around 10 o'clock each night. He then went straight to bed, got up early, and did it all again. George did this every day, seven days a week. The family restaurant was only closed three days a year—Christmas, Thanksgiving, and Good Friday—when his large Catholic family went to Mass. In short, he knew what hard work entailed, and this was what sold me.

When I told him, in that crowded clinic room that day, that I thought we could get him transplanted safely, he just smiled and nodded his head. His family shed tears, exchanged hugs, and clasped their hands together in silent prayer. I smiled, too, and put my hand on his shoulder. "Are you ready for this, George?" He took my hand off his shoulder and squeezed it tight. "Are *you* ready for this, Doc? Don't worry about me." His confidence startled me, his willingness to get in the boat with me and start rowing, to say to me in effect, "I'm not scared. Are you?"

And I wasn't. Each time I listed a patient for transplant—and there now have been hundreds—I saw myself as holding up an imaginary mirror and using it to reflect a patient's courage back to him, and together we would create a bond through our mutual leap of faith.

When George was transplanted after a short wait on our list, he became really sick, right out of the gate, the type of start to a transplant ICU course that my colleagues and I described somewhat callously as "trying to die sick."

George was essentially in full cardiac and respiratory arrest after the surgery when he arrived in the ICU room where I was waiting. That first night I stayed in his room for eighteen hours straight, changing ventilator settings and medications, waiting for something—anything—that would work. I left his room twice during that first day and night, once to go to the bathroom and once to eat microwave popcorn I had bummed off a nurse.

His condition didn't smooth out over the next two months. Almost every day and night, George presented to me every possible complication after a transplant: pneumonia, rejection, a perforated bowel, sepsis, and renal failure. Thrown in were intermittent and unpredictable episodes of unsustainable low blood pressure and instances where his lungs became so filled with mucous that the ventilator couldn't even force air into them.

When things got to this stage, I'd get called at home, dead asleep, to come in and do something to get George out of whatever crisis he was in. The nurses at his bedside had to call me in nearly every night for two months. It became so frequent that when I picked up the phone, the nurse would simply say, "David, it's George." I would then get out of bed and head to the hospital in a sleep-deprived fog, not able later to remember a minute of the drive. I then would take my now-familiar place at his bedside, racking my brain to think of some treatment to keep him alive until morning.

One night, after two months of this special kind of hell, George looked at me, as bleary-eyed and disoriented as I had ever seen a patient.

"I'm scared." He shook his head. "I can't die. I won't die."

I looked at him and held up that imaginary mirror I use to reflect a patient's courage back at him and said with all the determination I could muster as a young doctor of thirty-two, "You're not going to die. No one's dying. I've seen worse."

But I hadn't seen worse, or anything quite like it. What I thought I knew, this night and so many nights afterward, was that I could take a nasty, life-threatening disease with a bad set of facts, and help turn it around if I wanted to badly enough, if I tried hard enough. During the many nights George and I shared, we were like two men in a foxhole fighting like both of our lives depended on it. We were both always hoping the other guy had the "right stuff."

Finally, after three months in the hospital, George began to get better, at first imperceptibly, followed by a full-blown rally like only a twenty-something could muster. As he improved, he started to smile some, and so did I. He was going to make it. We had taken the risk together and won, due in part to my ability and perseverance, and mostly due to George's strength of character.

The day before he was to leave the hospital, I went to see him one last time. My sister Leslie, an attorney in New Orleans, was in town doing some work and I asked her to come to the hospital to meet him.

Leslie and I entered his room together, and as we walked in, George was getting ready to go, dressed in civilian clothes for the first time in over three months. After we went over some logistics regarding his follow-up care, he looked at Leslie and said, "You know, your brother is God." Leslie just laughed. But George and I weren't laughing. I knew why. We had risen up together, helped by the good work of our team, beating back whatever odds we faced. If it took belief in a higher force, so be it.

George's transplant was at the beginning of my twenty years on the front lines of transplant, when I was at my best. I looked back at my experience with George as having anchored me to the field, and the field to me. He was my star patient, the prototype of what transplant can do and what I could do using transplantation as an expression of my commitment to a cause for someone, to save a life.

George lived for eighteen years after his transplant. Soon after he returned home, he went back to the family restaurant, resuming his demanding work schedule and eventually running the business himself after his parents retired. He went on to have two beautiful children, their faces on the front of the cards he sent me every Christmas, cards I keep in a box near my desk. We spoke on the phone a few times a year, catching up on each other's lives, until he died.

When I have felt down over the years since George died, his many cards—over a dozen of them with pictures faithfully track his smiling children as they grew up—are a reminder of what we all have within us, of the magic that happens when we dig deep. When the will to survive exceeds the pain that is periodically delivered. This is transplantation at its absolute best, and why I would do anything in my power to make it work when patients were on my watch.

The problem is, transplantation does not always go well.

Twelve

Early in my time in Dallas, I got a close-up look at how events in transplantation—in life—can go so wrong that you can lose faith in other people and in yourself. Only three years after being recruited to start a new lung transplant program, I was trying to shut it down.

After doing a number of successful transplants the first two years, the following twelve months were a disaster. Complications, either during the donor procurement process or the operation itself, occurred in several consecutive patients. I knew regulatory agencies and insurance companies would threaten to put our program out of business if our outcomes didn't improve, and fast. Suddenly, our program's numbers were reflecting just how green we really were.

Regulatory bodies and private insurance companies measure the quality of a transplant program in terms of the percentage of patients who survive one year post-transplant. Patients want, and expect, to live much longer, but a one-year survival is a simple benchmark. A private organization, the Scientific Registry of Transplant Recipients, contracts with the U.S. Department of Health and Human Services to collect data about every transplant program in the country, which it publishes online. These data come out every six months, and every transplant program tracks its numbers closely in anticipation of these two times a year when its performance is quantitatively measured. Slipping to a one-year survival rate of around 80 percent or lower could put a program on the "watch list" of regulatory entities, which could cause insurance companies to cease sending insured patients to a center, which could ultimately put a program out of business.

These statistics are a validation of the program, a pass required to continue performing transplants. As if trying to save patients' lives weren't pressure enough, centers also have their survival rates published every six months. Many programs with talented doctors and surgeons simply fail to meet the benchmark, and regulatory agencies could shut them down—the equivalent of declaring bankruptcy.

This singular evaluation of the one-year survival rate is a flawed for several reasons. First, the numbers are too easy to manipulate and do not always accurately reflect how well patients truly do post-transplant. A program can keep a patient alive stuck on a mechanical ventilator or in a rehabilitation facility, barely mobile.

Second, focusing nearly exclusively on this one data point leaves out several other important metrics that could help to evaluate the quality of a transplant program, such as how long the average patient is hooked up to a ventilator or stays in the ICU or hospital, and how many patients develop problems with their other organs, such as their kidneys.

Finally, using only this metric discourages transplant programs from taking on any high-risk cases. Many programs operate under a "better safe than sorry" premise out of the fear of being shut down. This leaves the most high-risk patients, who are also the most vulnerable, with very few options when seeking a transplant center.

One day in early 1999, my third year as medical director in Dallas, I experienced the "big one": a complication so devastating that there was no way we could continue, even if we wanted to.

The donor call for this patient had come from one of our surgeons. I let the phone ring several times before I finally answered, still half asleep. As I began to speak to the surgeon, a close friend, I heard my answering machine pick up. I registered vaguely the fact that our conversation was being recorded, but it never occurred to me at the time that I would need that recording on the answering machine later.

For the surgeon and me, it was an easy decision that night: "She's listed for a left-lung transplant." "Yes, take the left lung, sounds fine." "Good, see you when you get out of the operating room." Even barely awake, I knew we were doing a left-lung transplant, as did the surgeon. My training had taught me to get the big things correct, no matter what.

The surgeon at the hospital removed the patient's left lung, expecting the procurement team to bring a left donor lung back to replace it. But the surgeon on our team that went to retrieve the donor lung brought back the right lung. In this case, the *wrong* lung. Suddenly, back in in our OR, there was a surplus of right lungs. We just didn't have a working left lung for our patient, Natalie.

Still in bed, I received a second call from the operating room. I couldn't make out what the caller was saying at first, but I did recognize the sounds of panic: people talking over one another, the rapid pace of their speech, the clanking sound of metal surgical instruments.

As soon as I understood what had happened, I sat bolt upright in bed. With a dull ache in my stomach and my heart pounding in my chest, I considered the inevitability that this woman would die. *This can't be happening.* We hadn't covered this type of scenario during my training, but it occurred to me we were going to need a lawyer.

Our team decided it would be best to do a right-lung transplant, since we had one available, leaving Natalie with no left lung. However, because of the fragility of a newly transplanted lung, it's vital to spread the blood flow over both. When only one is transplanted, it receives an overwhelming onslaught of pulmonary blood flow; it needs a counterpart to share the burden. In general, this scenario is unsustainable.

In the month that followed, Natalie remained in the ICU, clinging to life with little hope of survival. I saw her several times a day. It was a constant reminder of how we'd failed her. I played the night over and over in my mind. It felt like an open wound that refused to heal.

I had spoken with her family when things went so wrong the night of her transplant, and they knew her odds of survival. She was stuck in limbo, neither dead nor fully alive. We couldn't make her better, but the team wouldn't let her die, either, as that would have made final the mistakes we had made.

She ultimately died after a two-month slog in the ICU. We eventually did secure an attorney from a first-rate law firm in Dallas that had defended other doctors in the hospital, but never for anything quite so uniquely appalling.

For the next month, I spoke to the lawyers nearly every day—about as often as I spoke to Natalie's family. Eventually I'd have to find another job—to get away from the situation before we ended up in the newspaper. Sure, I had built the program over three years, but I was done. I'd gladly take a pay cut and start all over again at another hospital. I'd have to start back at the bottom of the ladder, but at least I'd be able to sleep at night.

I called a meeting with the surgical team and the leaders of our cardiothoracic surgery group so I could break the news to them. On that afternoon, I arrived late to the conference room on purpose. It was a clear winter day, and I noticed the sun looked like an orange fireball setting over the Texas skyline. The surgeons around the table stopped talking when I came in. They knew I was disenchanted, tired of poor outcomes, and sickened by the latest debacle.

But that wasn't entirely accurate. I was more than disenchanted; I was furious. Not everyone was at fault, but I was tired of the group trying to "manage" the situation, acting like the worst thing about what had happened was the negative PR it would bring to the hospital. A woman had lost her life, and no one could be bothered to take concrete steps to correct the problems. The hospital had no intention of getting rid of the surgeon who was responsible, despite his careless mistake. The incident would be "papered over"— the white coats had circled the wagons.

Everyone in the room was looking at me. I started right in.

"Well, no need to rehash the problems we've been having overall," I said. "But with this latest complication"—my face contorted with this euphemism—"I think it's safe to say that we should stop doing transplants here altogether."

The senior member of our group, Josh, who'd recruited me, spoke up first. He was six-foot-six and wore cowboy boots most of the time—even with his scrubs. He reminded me of John Wayne but seemed even more larger than life.

"What do you mean, 'stop doing transplants'? For how long?" His stare felt like it would bore a hole through my skull.

"Forever, would probably be the right call. But that's up to you. I won't be here. I'm leaving." I wanted to say, *"Listen, pal. You guys screwed up, and I'm not going to be here for the fallout."*

Then the lead transplant surgeon, Billy, a big-hearted, kind friend of mine, spoke up in his slow Texas drawl. He'd had no choice that night but to transplant Natalie's right lung.

"We can't do it without you," he said. "Who will replace you?"

"No one. You're not going to be able to find anyone to come here. Not after what's happened."

Josh looked lost in thought. His green eyes brightened suddenly. He pointed to Larry, a very good pulmonologist, who had been at the hospital a long time.

"What if you certified Larry?" The others at the table started robotically nodding in unison.

I was the only certified transplant doctor in the program, so for it to continue, they would either have to recruit someone already certified or certify one of the doctors already at our hospital. In the latter case, the doctor would need training to gain sufficient transplant experience, and that would take time. Transplant doctors weren't in plentiful supply then—and still aren't now.

I shook my head. "No disrespect to Larry, but he doesn't have any transplant experience." I was trying to state the facts plainly while also controlling my emotions. "The only time he's taken care of a transplant patient has been when I've been off—one week in the last three years. When I was on my honeymoon."

That's pretty dysfunctional, I thought.

Larry wrinkled his brow, trying to figure out what to say—or maybe think of a place to hide. His eyes avoided mine. It was clear suddenly that the others had already floated this possibility among themselves before the meeting; they must have known I was going to announce my departure, and now they were just trying to save their program and its revenues.

There was no way I could, in good conscience, certify Larry and just walk away, knowing patients would become casualties. Straightening up in my seat, I leaned forward and tapped my index finger on the table.

"I'm not certifying Larry. No way." I no longer cared whether my tone remained unemotional. "I'm not risking patients' lives, and my reputation, by endorsing him when he hasn't earned it. You don't need any more inexperience. You have plenty of it already."

With that, I walked out. In need of a new job. And a drink.

The program shut down soon after I left. Natalie's family received a confidential settlement out of court. As for the surgeon who'd made the mistake, there were no repercussions I'm aware of.

Thirteen

After Dallas, I accepted a position directing a well-established transplant program at the University of Alabama-Birmingham. UAB had a national reputation for excellence in all of the solid organ transplants: heart, lung, kidney, and liver. The lung program had great surgeons, especially an Australian guy named David McGiffin, with whom I would ultimately become rather close. Like many others, I admired not only his surgical skill but his can-do attitude and perpetual optimism. He was unfailingly congenial, and we shared a passion for transplant. In my entire career, I never worked with a better surgeon, or an individual with more integrity.

As a team, we got the lung transplant program rolling, transplanting patients who were considered to be at higher risk. Nonetheless, the outcomes were fantastic, and much of this was attributable to David's skill in the operating room. I did my best not to let him down with my work outside of the OR. We were so in sync that our conversations about prospective lung donors usually lasted about thirty seconds:

"Here's the deal, a lung with excellent function..."

"Yep. Sounds good. See you in the morning."

Between the two of us, there was no need for convincing or cajoling. No need for the "poker game," which is how some in our field describe the conversation/negotiation between physicians and surgeons about prospective donors. With us, it was just showtime. Looking at the waiting list, as I did often during the day, became a source of anticipation and pleasure because I knew these names would soon come off the list, one by one, as they got transplanted.

Soon after my arrival at UAB, my father received a liver transplant there. At the time of his transplant, I had been out of my training and in the field for five years. I was already accustomed to living the ups and downs with my patients, both the good outcomes and the bad, but I had lived through this as a doctor, not as a patient's family member. Big difference, as I would find out.

My father had been infected with hepatitis C from a blood transfusion he had received decades earlier, during one of his hip replacements. When he was diagnosed in 1998, it immediately occurred to me that he would likely need a liver transplant—and would soon enter my world of organ replacement.

One day in Birmingham, while talking to my father on the phone on my drive home from work, I brought up the possibility of a liver transplant. His response was lackluster.

"No, I don't think so. If it's my time, then so be it." I swallowed hard, keeping my eyes on the line of traffic in front of me. My father was controlling and determined with most things in life, but when it came to his own health, he was nihilistic. This was bewildering to those of us close to him, because his resignation was so out of character, so contrary to his normal grit and self-assuredness.

In the wake of his hepatitis C diagnosis, my dad's health deteriorated. Over several months he lost a lot of weight and was ultimately too weak to get out of bed most days. When I visited him at his home in Colorado in 2000, I was struck by the orange glow of his jaundiced skin—a classic sign of end-stage liver failure. His days were limited. Though my dad had never been one to share his feelings, I could tell he knew he was dying, and he finally told me, on a gray winter day in the mountains, that he wasn't ready to die.

And neither was I. Transplant was his last hope, and during that visit, I made a strong sales pitch. He agreed—reluctantly—to at least explore the possibility.

By 2001, his condition had progressed to the point that he urgently needed the transplant. Back then, almost all transplants were performed on people younger than sixty; programs occasionally took older patients, but never one as old as my father, who was sixty-eight. According to convention, he was too old for a transplant. And in addition to the problems from his advanced liver disease, his mobility was now limited due to a limp resulting from his multiple orthopedic operations. To transplant physicians, he looked like a bad candidate for major surgery, even a lifesaving one. The concern was that he would be unable to get up and walk soon after the surgery—a key component to postoperative recovery.

Despite the apparent obstacles, I pitched the idea to Bob Murphy, who ran Birmingham's liver transplant program. I had shared with Bob my dad's condition earlier, but only as a friend confiding in a friend, never in the context of asking for help. This time, during one of our bike rides together, I communicated the urgency of the situation.

"Bob, my dad's liver disease is getting worse," I told him. "He's going down quickly. I think I want you to see him for a transplant evaluation."

"Sure thing," Bob said. "How old is he?"

"Sixty-eight." I glanced over at him to try to read his face. We pedaled along in silence.

Is he working out the right way to say no to a friend? We rounded a large bend in the road.

Finally, he said simply, "Sure, I'll see him. I'll set it up."

I looked skyward, smiling with relief.

A few weeks later, Bob met with my father and found him engaging. More importantly, Bob had faith that my father could get through the operation. So, despite Dad's age and condition, Bob put him on the waiting list.

When I heard the good news, I felt guilty—for just a heartbeat. I knew how transplant worked: it's a zero-sum game. When one person gets an organ, it usually means another person won't, at least at that moment, and the next person on the list might not survive while waiting for their turn.

Is my father less deserving than younger patients—people with their entire lives ahead of them? Will he now be the reason a mother or father with little kids doesn't receive a lifesaving transplant? More to the point, is this fair? I had used my privilege and access to get my father on the waiting list— was this the medical equivalent of insider trading? Maybe, maybe not. I'll never know for sure. But the situation got me thinking about the ethics of the transplant recipient evaluation criteria, and whether it is ever, or even usually, equitable.

I learned the answer then, but I would confirm it again and again over the course of my career. In the transplant world, we simply do not distribute access and information equitably. As in all aspects of American healthcare, racial and socioeconomic disparities pervade all phases of the transplant journey. No matter which organ someone needs, whether it's a heart, lung, kidney, or liver, there are baked-in inequalities that impact the access of certain groups to get on the waiting list. Beyond that, as I came to see, these factors also influence one's ability to, once listed, actually receive a transplant, and achieve an outcome comparable to that of people who are white or enjoy greater socioeconomic status. Our transplant group at Stanford contributed to this research in terms of the heart and lung transplant.

We found, for instance, that black heart transplant recipients had a higher mortality than white patients, even after adjusting for the baseline risk factors for group before transplant. The same was true in lung transplant, although we found that the survival differences by race had not been observed in the more recent transplant era. Apart from survival after a transplant, the access to transplant and the ability to get on a center's waiting list, is also diminished for non-white people, regardless of which organ—heart, lung, kidney, or liver—is needed.

The research is clear: the color of your skin can affect your outcome following transplantation. As far as we know, this is not because of overt racial discrimination on the part of the practitioners—although I suspect it is nonetheless a form of unconscious bias—but certainly there is unequal access to healthcare in general, especially the complex kind like transplantation.

In transplant the disparities become more obvious because we are constantly making subjective decisions in selecting who is (and is not) a candidate. This perhaps sets us apart from other aspects of healthcare practitioners, who must treat everyone who walks through the door. The patients are essentially selecting themselves. Not in transplant. We pick our patients by sitting around a conference table as a group, looking at objective data accompanied by subjective judgments that are surely influenced heavily, perhaps unconsciously, by each of our life experiences.

This is the disparity for people who need a transplant, but there is also presumably an impact of race in terms of the propensity to consent for organ donation.

You can see grief from all the way down the hall.

At the end of the long hospital corridor is the ICU waiting room—the center of misery at most hospitals.

As I get closer, I see a family, holding on to each other, huddled together. An older woman is crying—chanting—"Oh my Lord, oh my Lord. Oh my Lord, *why* my Lord?"

It was my second year in Birmingham. The transplant program was going well, and on this night, there was a potential organ donor in the medical ICU. The local organ procurement organization had called me, asking me, since the donor was in our hospital, if I could come and assess the donor's quality. This entailed evaluating the brain-dead patient's chest X-ray, lab studies, and medical history.

When I arrived at his bedside, I quickly assessed the situation and found a disturbing but all-too-familiar story. A young black man named Donald, with no past medical problems, had suffered a gunshot wound to the head. Allegedly the incident had occurred over an argument about something no one could identify. When the paramedics had found Donald, he was barely breathing. Given the extent of his injury, it was amazing that he had survived at all. He was quickly intubated and brought to UAB hospital. After several hours of attempts to resuscitate him, the team declared him brain dead earlier that day.

I approached the organ procurement organization coordinator at Donald's bedside. This was a delicate business.

"Has the family given consent?"

"They haven't said yes but hadn't said no either," she said. "They're waiting to talk with their pastor and some other family members."

It is a gross understatement to say that a family's decision to donate is a big one, and their loved one has usually not made clear their intentions before tragedy struck. This made it that much tougher to "do the right thing"—or even know what the right thing is.

After looking at the details of Donald's medical situation, I was satisfied his lungs would be acceptable to use for one of our wait-listed patients, provided of course the family decided to consent to donate.

As I walked out of the ICU, I took out my waiting list, scanning the names, looking at the patients' sizes and blood types, trying to find a good fit for Donald's lungs. The double doors swung open, and as I was moving quickly down the hall by the waiting room, I heard a voice, an unusually deep baritone.

"Doctor, can I speak with you?"

I glanced up, unsure if the voice was directed at me.

I looked over at a tall, well-dressed man standing by the family, looking straight at me. "Are you Donald's doctor?" the man asked.

I stuck out my hand, and we shook. He told me he was the family's pastor and had known Donald since he was a boy—the same one whom I had just been hovering over, evaluating the quality of his organs for harvest. The pastor may have seen a little boy from the church pews when he looked into that room in the ICU, whereas I only saw two lungs—which we needed desperately for one of the long-suffering, fragile patients on my flimsy piece of paper.

"I am a lung transplant doctor here, and I was seeing Donald, because he is...umm...might be.... Well, he is brain dead, and sometimes in this situation...umm...when this happens, the tragedy, families choose organ donation." The pastor didn't say anything as he quietly sized me up. Then he spoke.

"So you are not trying to save Donald. You are interested in his organs." He said it as a matter of fact, unblinking, seemingly not judging, but making it clear the time for bullshitting was over.

"Well, no...I mean, yes. While he is considered dead according to the definition of the state law, it's entirely the family's choice if he becomes an organ donor. Or not."

"But his heart is still beating?" he asked.

"Yes."

The pastor thought for a moment. "But he's dead?"

"Yes." I decided to stick to yes or no answers.

"Tell me this, Doctor…"

"It's Dr. Weill." I stuck out my hand again. "David Weill," I smiled as warmly as I could. "David." *Sir, you can trust me.*

He took my hand, slowly but with conviction. And then let my hand linger in his for an uncomfortable period of time.

"*If* he is dead," as though it were merely a theory I was floating, "did you do everything you could to save him?"

I was knocked off balance by his calling my professionalism into question "Well, yes…I mean, I wasn't his doctor. But yes. The doctors in the ICU did everything they could." He looked at me and then back at the family, who had stopped talking and were watching the two of us. He had an audience.

"Are you sure?" I thought he might be testing me.

"Yes, I'm sure." He paused, waiting for me to elaborate. I didn't.

"Then let's go talk with the family."

I sat down in a row of chairs across from them—Donald's mother, aunt, and two sisters. The pastor stood behind Donald's mother, with a hand on her shoulder.

"Are you trying to save my baby?" Donald's mother asked.

"I am so sorry about what happened to your son," I said. "I wish I could save him, but I can't. He's gone." I paused. "I'm a transplant doctor, and I'm here to see if Donald would be a suitable donor for transplant."

Their tears began to flow, the family understandably having difficulty with the stark reality I had presented. His mother stiffened, clenched her jaw, and asked, "If his heart is still beating, how can he be dead?"

One of his sisters chimed in. "He's not dead. Donald's not dead."

I had heard this before from a prospective donor's family. I agreed it was hard to understand. Brain death has a medical and legal definition: the complete and irreversible loss of brain function. But families see the heart beating, and air going in and out of the lungs via the mechanical ventilator, and think that is still life.

But it's not—it's only the appearance of life made possible by the assistance of life support. In fact, if organ donation is not a possibility, care providers can stop life support without the family's consent.

Then death would be clear to patients' families. But it was very clear to me now that Donald was dead. And yes, I wanted the family to realize this and agree to donate his organs. I had a waiting list in my pocket full of names of people who needed his healthy lungs, people I knew, people I felt responsible for. And I knew Donald couldn't use his any longer.

"Ma'am, I know this is a lot to take in, and I am reluctant to ask, but I wonder if you can find a place in your heart to help these other people, some of them my own patients, who need a transplant to live." I waited for her reaction but there was none.

"Can you, and Donald, give this gift?" I asked. She then started crying again and stood up to hug the pastor.

"NO, NO, how can this be? They want my baby's organs!" I stood and put my hand on her shoulder.

"I am so sorry." I had nothing better to say, so I kept saying it over and over, how sorry I was, how tough it is. She composed herself and looked me right in the eye.

"You know what you can do?" I waited, hopeful she would consent to donation.

"You can go back in there and save my son. *That's* what you can do."

I nodded, stepping back, recoiling, wanting to give her emotional space but also wanting to get out of there. Her pain, mixed with her justifiable anger, was rushing out of her, accelerating, and slapping me in the face. I backpedaled.

"Take care, ma'am. I'll come back and see you later."

Then she expressed her rage. "No need to come back. We aren't donating Donald's organs. He's not done with them yet." Her voice was loud and clear now. It echoed around the waiting room and down the hall, even catching the attention of the elderly volunteer in the waiting room some fifty feet away.

As I walked away from the ICU, I thought, *How can she not agree to donate? How can she not agree to help all these dying people—my dying people?*

Then it occurred to me. *Trust. She doesn't have any trust.*

It wasn't disdain, although it might have sounded that way. Her distrust was not about me specifically—I didn't think, anyway—but I was a white doctor in a white coat, telling her that her son was dead, when all could see his heart was beating strong.

No, she didn't trust my message—what I was asking. She heard, "I want to take that strong heart, and those lungs, too, and maybe a kidney or two, and put them in someone else who is more important than your son."

This mother didn't trust me, or the medical establishment, to do the right thing. I sensed her perception was that we could save her son, but we chose not to.

Just then I thought of Tuskegee and its infamous "Study of Untreated Syphilis in the African American Male." She knew what had happened, I suspected. We in the medical field had forgotten about it or tried to forget. We had moved on, but she hadn't. She didn't trust us, the white medical people, so there would not be any signed consent.

This is what she was saying to me.

And because of distrust, I wasn't going to be able to take a name off my list. Not tonight.

To make it onto a waiting list, there is also something subtle going on, not as obvious as the color of your skin, how much money you have, or the quality of your health insurance. It has to do with who you are and how you present yourself.

My father, for example, was a well-spoken academician with the publications, titles, honors, and professorships that go along with a prolific career. He earned every bit of it, as an immigrant who came to this country with no money, unable to speak the language, in essence, a war refugee. He was a man who had a lot to be admired. As my father was being evaluated for a possible transplant, "sized up," if you will, by people with similar life experience—academic achievers, those who sought and received awards, those with scholarly publications—would it be any surprise if the doctors looked at him as "one of them"? It would be nearly impossible not to see him as a doctor, just like them. When I evaluated whether to list a patient for transplant, I found myself doing the same thing with potential recipients, spending an hour sizing them up. Perhaps this one was gifted with a winning personality, a spirit that was contagious, or—I am reluctant to admit—was a "success" in life, as measured by society. Sometimes, when it comes to replacing an organ, it can come down to how you present yourself and whether the transplant team "likes" you. In effect, the social skills you learned early in life can now save your life.

Partly because of me, my father was able to get in front of the people with the power to save his life before it was too late. And because of me, and also because of his professional background as an accomplished physician-scientist, these people perceived him as a person in need of a liver, rather than a data point with the potential to negatively skew the program's survival statistics because of his relatively advanced age.

As mentioned earlier, UAB had a strong liver program, having done some of the earliest and best work in the field. The transplant center there did well over four hundred solid organ transplants each year with excellent outcomes.

I did feel twinges of guilt for using my connections to help get my father transplanted. But I wanted him transplanted any way I could. I tried to focus on the possibility that he would have been transplanted without my help, which is more likely today, since the comfort level in the field with transplanting older patients has increased.

Once, in the early stages, when my father was just beginning to consider getting a transplant, he'd told me he would never let me donate part of my liver to him in a split liver transplant. The procedure is used to save the patient if it is not likely that a cadaveric (deceased) donor can be found in time, as well as in less dire circumstances, when a family member or friend chooses to become a donor.

"Don't worry. I'm not offering," I'd joked at the time, using humor to deflect the seriousness of the subject. "With my alcohol consumption, I'm going to need all the liver I've got."

"Good," he'd replied. "Maybe you could just help get me the transplant the normal way." He knew I could try, but we didn't want to directly confront it for a good reason: Neither of us wanted him to "owe" me for something so big. In a relationship that wasn't built on showing our inner emotions, I knew my father could not handle me helping him in such a profound way.

As my father's need for transplant became an impending reality, my role in his life weaved between son, advocate, teacher, and guide. I'd gone through this process with hundreds of other patients, but the emotional stakes were different now that the patient was someone with whom I had a long and complex personal relationship.

Given that I was a relatively unengaged student early on, I doubt that either my friends or family could have predicted that I would have been in the position to help my father in this way, but here we were. No one could have foreseen that one day I would have the opportunity to help save my father's life—with a big assist from the UAB liver transplant team, of course. If it felt wrong to pull strings, it would have felt that much more wrong to let him die without giving him the second chance he deserved.

Fourteen

T he donor call came just a few months after my father
was listed for transplant. I was off work on a Sunday,
watching football, when the phone rang.

Dr. Bob Murphy, the liver surgeon, cut right to the
chase. "Hey David, where's your father?"

"Colorado. Got something for him?" I stood up and
started my usual pre-transplant pacing. Sitting still was not
my strong suit anyway, but it was impossible when it came
time for a transplant, regardless of whether it was one of my
patients or my own father.

"Yeah, there's a liver that I think would work for him.
Motorcycle accident. Young guy." My heart raced.

After hanging up with Bob, I called my father at home.
"Hey, Dad. What's up?"

"Nothing. Watching a game." Not surprisingly, he was
also watching football. He sounded far away, tired, and weak.

When I was growing up, my father and I watched every
Saints game together. I'd sit close to the television and my
father would sit in his regular chair, sometimes reading the
newspaper at the same time, sometimes sipping a beer. At
halftime, we would go outside and throw the football—
but only after I'd put on a Saints jersey and helmet he had

given me for my birthday. I would run out for passes and my father nearly always overthrew me, no matter how fast I ran. He told me I needed to speed up, learn to run faster. I'd go get the ball, run back to him, sweat pouring everywhere, and give him the ball. I'd then line up again, determined this time to run fast enough to catch his pass.

I hesitated at first, then launched right in. "Look, I think they have a liver for you." Nothing. I could tell he was preoccupied with the game. I raised my voice a bit and tried again.

"Hey, I think your transplant is going to happen tonight." Still no response.

Now I was standing, pacing again. Even louder this time, I said, "Dad, looks like the transplant's going to happen! You need to come here! Right away! Call the airplane people!" We had set up a private plane charter for when we got the call, and we needed to give them some notice. The clock was beginning to run.

"You mean...now?" He sounded annoyed. "Can it wait until after the game?"

I couldn't believe it. *Why don't we just make it two weeks from Friday? Would that be more convenient?*

"No, it cannot wait until after the game," I said, enunciating each word slowly, with increasing impatience. *Fuck— Can it wait until after the game?!* This was so like my dad, wanting to do everything, including his liver transplant, on his own time, and on his own terms. He was controlling, but also probably scared.

If he was going to get the liver, he had to hurry to the hospital. And he was halfway across the country. I'd been like a broken record when it came to my own patients over the years, telling them to always have a bag ready, explaining that when the call came, they should move quickly, but not rush. "No car accidents," I'd tell them. "It really puts a damper on the whole transplant thing."

It was important to me to help patients feel comfortable during these high-stakes, anxiety-inducing situations. To accommodate patients who lived out of town, we could give them about four hours to get to the hospital. My father was *way* out of town, though—two thousand miles away. He needed to get a move on.

After what felt like several weeks but was only several hours, my parents—and the family cat, Logan—landed at the Birmingham airport. It was two in the morning when I picked them up, and we headed straight for the hospital. I made a conscious effort to drive a normal speed, heeding my own advice.

Within the hour, my dad was admitted to the hospital and my mother went to check into the hotel where they would stay once he was discharged. Everything, and everyone, was in place.

In my father's hospital room, both of us quickly got bored waiting for his new liver. We were staring at the small TV mounted on the hospital room wall, my father in the bed and me in a chair close by. It was just a few days after 9/11, and the TV was playing continuous loops of World Trade Center footage.

"Hurry up and wait. It's always been that way," my father said, rolling his eyes. "Medical care…not exactly efficient."

"It always slows down at the donor hospital," I said. "The team went out only an hour ago—I bet we have another hour until we hear if the organs are okay."

"Seems to take longer than it should." Given my father's German heritage, his love of efficiency and precision, waiting around was not a strength of his. "We'll just have to watch some more depressing news," he said.

Focusing our attention on the falling Twin Towers and the crying families was a sad distraction from the difficult conversation we could have been having.

After another hour, a transporter finally came to wheel my dad to surgery. When he lined up the gurney next to the hospital bed, my father asked if he could stand up and get on himself—one last attempt to maintain control and avoid seeming as sick as he was. Unfortunately for him, the transporter politely declined. It was against hospital policy. My father reluctantly conceded.

With his orthopedic difficulties and an abdomen filled with fluid due to his liver failure, even sliding from the bed onto the gurney was difficult. He tried to do it himself before accepting help from the transport person and myself, while grimacing the entire time. We finally got him situated. He straightened his hospital gown and heaved a sigh.

"Okay, all set?" the transporter asked.

"I guess," my father replied. He didn't appear frightened, just inconvenienced. As he was being wheeled out, he took my mother's hand, gave it a quick squeeze, and then let go.

My mother stayed behind in the room, and I walked beside the gurney as my father was wheeled down the hall. When we got to the pre-op area, where the transporter would need to take him back, my father and I stared at each other, both of us struggling with what to say. Finally, he broke the awkwardness. Eyebrows arched, he had a smile on his face.

"Well, is there anything else you want to know from me?"

"No, I don't think so. I think I'm good." *I want to know more—so much more. What's most important to you in life? Your work? Your family? What was it like being run out of your home country as a small boy? Were you scared? Did you feel "other"? And maybe most important: What do you think of me? Are you proud of me?*

I didn't ask any of these questions, or anything else. I was closed up, stoic, in keeping with my medical training.

With that, my father was wheeled through the automatic doors into the holding area. I watched the doors close, then stood there staring for a while.

As I walked back to my mother waiting in the hospital room, I thought, *Is this the last time I will ever see my father?*

And how we had just botched our goodbye.

Fifteen

My dad recovered from transplant without a hitch—aside from thinking that Colin Powell was in the hospital room next to his (a hallucinatory effect from the pain medication). His five-day stay in the hospital would have been considered short for any patient, but for a sixty-eight-year-old, it was astonishing.

He and my mother were staying at a nearby hotel, the choice of many of our out-of-town patients requiring frequent visits to the transplant clinic.

During those first few weeks, my father didn't spend much time learning about his medications. Instead, he relied on my mother to lay them out for him and tell him what to take. It frustrated me to see him be so nonchalant about the gift he'd been given. *Does he truly not care? Or is he frightened? Is being so blasé about the whole thing his only way to handle the fear and loss of control?* I was left guessing, since he wasn't one to tell me, or anyone else, what was on his mind. But I knew this for sure: though he may have been reluctant to get his transplant, it was too late for apathy. The liver, one might say, was out of the barn.

Giving up on discussing his medications for the time being, I was watching TV with my father a few days later when a different issue rose in my mind. I needed to remind him about writing a letter to his donor's family. We'd discussed the idea before when I'd explained how important it was in helping the recipient process, the tremendous impact of the donor's decision. Transplant program social workers were normally the ones who encouraged patients to do this, simply to say thank you and acknowledge the selflessness of the act. But in my dad's case I was wearing many hats, acting as transplant physician, social worker, and drill sergeant.

I asked my father if he needed help with the letter. I assumed he wasn't going to write it unless I kept after him about it.

"I'll get to it at some point," he said, as he watched the news.

"You need to do it soon. It's important." There was no protocol on how soon after the transplant these letters should be written, but I knew the longer he waited, the less likely he was to do it.

He clicked the TV off and turned to me. "What's with you? You've been at this all night. Mind your own business."

To me, it *was* my business. I didn't necessarily need him to direct gratitude toward me, but I did need him to show some gratitude for transplantation, to show some respect for how difficult it is and how much skill it takes to do it right. I was conflating the success of transplant, anyone's transplant, with my success as a person. In retrospect, this wasn't healthy and, ultimately, it would prove to be unsustainable.

Yet even if my father's transplant didn't transform him, it did change me. I became even more enamored with the mystique of transplant, the wonder of it all. I no longer saw it as just medical therapy for people who needed it but considered my job to be something more sacred—even a spiritual calling. I hoped to do more than excel; the responsibility now consumed me in a way it never had before.

The idea that I could play a part in saving a life—especially that of my own father—felt like a power surge within me, and that motivated me even more.

I knew intellectually that transplant was a risky business, filled with uncertainties and potential complications. But emotionally I refused to accept it. I was chasing an impossible standard, deluded that I could give every patient the perfect transplant. In my way of thinking then, I could control outcomes if I just worked hard enough and smart enough. I wanted to hit a home run every time I went to bat.

Sixteen

After a few years in Birmingham, I started to look for other job opportunities. My motivation to make a change was not due to what was happening at the hospital—things were going well—but rather that Jackie and I wanted to be in a different part of the country. Like many young couples without kids, we were looking for a bit more excitement. Although Birmingham was a perfectly nice place to live and we had met some wonderful people there, we both felt that it was time to go. When I mentioned to my old mentor Marty Zamora that I was looking to change jobs, he said, "Why don't you come back to Denver?" So we did. It was that simple. I had great memories of my training period there and loved Colorado.

When I started working in Denver, things were much the same as I had left them six years earlier, but I was struck by how much I had changed. Not yet forty, I had already been in charge of two transplant programs and had gained all the experiences these programs had to offer: the responsibility, the power to make the tough decisions, and the recognition from patients and colleagues when things went well. I knew I wanted all these things. But when I got back to Colorado, it was Marty's show, and rightly so. I either had to accept this or leave to lead another program.

In the meantime, we had success that was, in many ways, intoxicating. We had four great surgeons, including Dr. Grover, who had trained me and with whom I got along well. And Marty and I made a great team. We were built the same way: intense, dedicated, and self-assured (which might be an understatement). Like an ego-driven older brother-younger brother relationship, we would occasionally snipe at one another and compete. Despite this, the team produced outstanding results, performing close to one hundred transplants in the four years I was there—without losing a single patient during the hospitalization immediately following the transplant. I have no way of knowing if this has ever been done elsewhere, but I had never heard of, let alone experienced, these kinds of results—and I have not since. Apparently, a team of rivals can at times be effective.

My success at work was not matched at home, however. I had not left enough time in my day for Jackie. She didn't complain, because she understood that the long hours were part of the job. I was wrapped up in my work, and my family bore the brunt of that neglect.

When Hannah was born, in the hospital next door to where I was working, I took no time off and would split my time, going back and forth from Jackie's hospital room to my patients across the street. By the time we took Hannah home from the hospital, I was already back at work, listening to my colleagues saying things like, "Get back to work. Having babies is women's work." Just a few hours after Hannah was born, one of my mentors in Denver said he was glad to see me at work. "It's not like you delivered the baby."

Seventeen

In 2005, Stanford called to offer me a job. They were one of the first hospitals to become involved in thoracic transplantation, but their lung program had fallen on tough times—a shrinking number of patients being transplanted and too many poor outcomes. As a result, the program had been placed on a probationary status; if things didn't improve, the regulatory agencies could shut down the program. Perhaps even more likely, the insurance companies would simply stop allowing their insured patients to receive transplants there, which would essentially kill the program. As at many struggling transplant programs, the hospital administrators were trying to evaluate what to do next.

Looking back on Stanford's decision to continue its lung transplant program, and the many hospital leaders I have consulted for about it, begs a fundamental question: Why do hospitals want transplant programs? To help people. To save lives. Mostly. But not exclusively.

If you are a hospital, transplant makes you cool. Just like a guy who wants a fancy car, hospitals want to be hip, too. And transplant is hip. It is a sexy therapy, dramatic and newsworthy. Transplant is different from the more mundane delivery of healthcare, like birthing babies or fixing broken arms. It's a differentiator.

There are a few of these differentiators—you can tell what they are by what the major hospitals choose to advertise. Cancer centers. The latest in neuroscience breakthroughs. And, of course, the consistent winner: cardiac care.

Why do hospitals want differentiators? Because medicine is a business. Most obviously because a differentiator by definition means that you are providing something not everyone can offer, in this case a specific form of medical therapy. Equally important, advertising a specialized form of care signals to the patients/consumers that if they can trust us to do the more complex procedures, they should trust us to do the routine stuff. Doing appendectomies can't be as hard as doing transplants, right? If you can do transplants, you can presumably do appendectomies.

I am oversimplifying, but hospitals don't make much profit by providing routine, necessary, medical care. This is not to say they don't want the routine business. They do— it rounds out the full-service commitment many hospitals have, and it serves a community purpose. But the areas that have high profit margins are the differentiators.

I don't want to leave the impression that hospital administrators and hospital boards of directors are in the game exclusively to make money. Mostly they are not. However, they are running a business, and accordingly, they make business decisions. This should not come as a surprise, nor should the concept be lost on patients or on staff. It's as universal as the bad food in hospital cafeterias.

In September 2005, as I was trying to decide whether to take the job at Stanford, Hurricane Katrina hit New Orleans. Watching the coverage on television was crushing, reminding me of 9/11, when none of us could shut off the news.

My hometown was in turmoil in the days after the storm, its people in despair, neighborhoods washed away, buildings that had been there for centuries burned to the ground. My sister Leslie and her daughter, Katy, had evacuated to Atlanta as the storm approached, and finally to Denver to stay with us.

This hurricane affected me viscerally, as it did so many others who loved the city. I needed to understand how something so tragic, on such a massive scale, could have happened, and though I didn't have any formal religion in my life at that point, I turned to the Bible.

Like most undertakings, I went all in. I decided to read it cover to cover, both the Old and New Testament. I used a daily Bible reader that guided me through the entire text in a year. Each morning, I read the assigned passages for that day as soon as I got up, highlighting certain sections or writing notes in the margins.

I took great interest in what I was reading and was amazed at how little human struggles have changed. I was comforted by the notion that what I grappled with in my own life was much the same trials people had faced hundreds and even thousands of years ago. I read until I finished the entire Bible. And then I read it again the next year, and the year after. That was my Katrina experience.

In the months leading up to my accepting the Stanford position, my father expressed his disappointment about my plan.

"Moving again?" he would ask. "How many jobs are you going to have in your career? I had one and did pretty well at it."

Not me. The only way I knew how to work was to take risks, to do things differently. My father liked routine and found comfort in it. For me, routine was the enemy, to be avoided at all costs. I had felt the sameness of my job in Denver sinking in. I relished the thought of a new program, a new challenge, a new part of the country.

"Dad, it's Stanford, for heaven's sake. It's a great position—I'm being asked to lead one of the original transplant programs in the country, not to work in an urgent care clinic somewhere."

"Well, you might as well be. Plus, the cost of living is ridiculous out there. You're going to go broke."

Ultimately, despite my father's misgivings, I decided to take the job, and my family packed up to move further west.

Even as a grown man, I sought my parents' approval—especially my father's. My mother gave hers unconditionally. But my father's unwillingness to support my taking the position at Stanford cast a pall over our move to California. In fact, my attitude upon starting the job was both disappointment and defiance toward my father: *Hey, fuck off. I'll show you that this was the right move.* At the time, these were my default emotions when facing most challenges.

By then I had ten years of transplant experience and was, theoretically, at the top of my game. I was past making rookie mistakes, and my learning curve had flattened. Though I wasn't eager to uproot my family, heading this lung transplant program was exciting. Remaking myself every few years was my modus operandi, and this opportunity was fresh and filled with potential. I was ready to go.

PART TWO

*Each of us, however old, is still an undergraduate
in the school of experience. When a man thinks he
has graduated, he becomes a public menace.*
—John Chalmers DaCosta

One

Dog. Shit. Tired. Walking right into a closed-door kind of tired. The kind of tired that feels like a wet blanket is wrapped around the brain. Up three nights in a row evaluating lung donors from places I can't even remember. Could have been Fresno. No, San Jose. Maybe Modesto. Maybe not. They were somewhere, their misfortune leading to someone else's incredible fortune. People I didn't know who were giving a gift to people I did know, patients I desperately wanted to save.

One of the donors was a teenager who had been thrown out of the bed of a pickup truck going seventy miles an hour, scattering beer cans and body parts all over the road. Another young man, this one in his twenties, had skied headfirst without a helmet into a tree on a Lake Tahoe downhill run. The third donor, a guy in his mid-fifties, had experienced a cerebral bleed while in bed with someone who wasn't his wife.

These three men had not likely woken up that morning thinking that by nightfall they would become organ donors.

But the people who received their gift, the gift of life, had woken up that very same morning wondering if that day would be *their* day.

I couldn't wait to get to the hospital each morning. Back then, going to work was easy—I never had to set an alarm clock, and my first thought was never, *Don't want to do it— not interested today.* I liked a lot of it—the pace, the rhythm, the feeling of doing something that was consequential.

When I arrived at the hospital, I would go to see my patients who had received transplants in the last week and were still in the ICU, trying to breathe with their new lungs. They were waiting for the magic to happen, for the moment when the brain realizes the organs it's just received can provide the oxygen it desperately needs.

Then I'd be off to the outpatient clinic, seeing twenty patients, all at various post-transplant stages—some just a month out, others a year, a few even ten years and still going strong. After the clinic, I'd have a meeting with some of the hospital financial staff, who loved transplant as much as I did, but for different reasons. In late afternoon I had more hospital rounds, and then I'd head home for dinner with my family.

But right now, it was 6:30 a.m. and I was ready.

Jackie was less than thrilled with the move to Palo Alto. Our two daughters were young at the time—Hannah was three and Ava just a couple months old—and this was Jackie's third move for my career. Ambitious and ego driven, I expected my family to follow along. I was suffering from a hero complex that made me want to fix everything—especially broken transplant programs.

When I had met Jackie in 1996, she was working as a nurse. I finally understood what people meant by "Midwestern values." She was tough, smart, and had the strongest character of anyone I had ever met. And she was strikingly beautiful—tall, blonde, blue eyes. A move to a tony part of California was not going to worry her much, and despite her reluctance, Jackie organized everything for our move without a single complaint. Having spent her childhood on a farm in rural Iowa—rising early, feeding the pigs, and even driving farm equipment, starting at age fourteen—she was not one to shy away from hard work. When I was fourteen, I was riding my bike in the French Quarter, taking in the smell, sights, and sounds so much part of the New Orleans tapestry. The two of us could not have grown up in more different environments.

When we got to California, my work at the hospital kept me busy around the clock. The program had not kept up with modern transplant practices. In fact, it appeared the hospital had intentionally kept the program as small as possible. In the transplant business, a small transplant program is usually a failing transplant program. In a small program, the team just doesn't get enough experience to perform well. It would be akin to flying with a team of pilots who hardly ever actually fly airplanes. I'd take a different airline. Patients who might have considered going to Stanford for their transplant instead went to a different hospital.

In the year prior to my arrival, the team had performed a total of only eleven lung transplants, with only about half of the patients making it to the first year following their surgery. Now I understood why.

When I interviewed for the position, the hospital CEO asked me if I thought there was any point in continuing to offer lung transplants at Stanford. Not exactly a reassuring question to ask the person interviewing for the head of transplant, but not unreasonable either. The poor outcomes had even drawn the kind of attention transplant programs didn't want—from regulators and insurance companies who demanded improvements, the worst potential consequence being shut down altogether.

I didn't think the program was a lost cause and said as much in my interview. In fact, I told the CEO something she probably already knew: the surgical team was a group of the most experienced physicians in the country and had been in on the ground floor when lung transplant became a reality in the mid- to late 1980s. The surgical team was not the problem—it was the medical team responsible for the post-operative care. I was confident I could shore up that side of things.

My new job was simple. I needed to do two things: increase the number of patients transplanted at Stanford and improve their survival after receiving the transplant. Easy to say, harder to do. This was what I was recruited to do, and what I most wanted to do—fix the program so we could then fix people.

I first had to address the program personnel. I needed to get doctors, nurses, nurse practitioners, pharmacists, and social workers on board with my vision for the program. To recruit people costs money, so I spent considerable time convincing the hospital financial staff that new recruitments were necessary. I ended up developing a close working relationship with the hospital administrators responsible for the transplant program, and they became close collaborators with me in rebuilding the program.

Once the team was in place, and with no detail overlooked, I started where I always did: looking at every aspect of the program and changing practices that seemed to be outdated or substandard. For example, the long form that referring physicians were required to fill out for us to consider a patient for a transplant needed to be revamped. The current form gave the impression that we were protecting our castle from outside invaders. Anyone who has seen a doctor knows how the medical field uses forms extensively, but what I discovered in Stanford's transplant program was beyond anything I'd ever seen—a lengthy packet that was both cumbersome and unnecessary. We would eventually find out what we needed to know in our evaluation process once the patient came to be seen at Stanford.

Another example involved the social workers preventing patients from being considered for a transplant simply because their living circumstances were "less than ideal." Or even worse—age restrictions and other strict criteria that were more than a conservative approach. They were clearly outdated.

I also noted inefficiencies in the way patients were scheduled for clinic. A patient was scheduled at 9:00 a.m., for instance, and then another at 1:00 p.m., and another at 3:00 p.m. This resulted in trapping the entire multidisciplinary transplant team—the doctors, the nurses, the nurse practitioners, the social workers, the dietitians, the pharmacists—in the clinic for hours, waiting around for the next patient to arrive.

I changed the schedule so all patients came in at 9:00 a.m., after which each team member would see a patient in one of six rooms, do their evaluation, and then rotate to the next room. It looked like a game of musical chairs, but it worked smoothly. Using this schedule, each patient got the attention they needed from each of us, and the transplant team could complete clinic visits and then get on with their day, whether they were seeing sick patients in the hospital, doing administrative tasks, tending to the electronic medical record, or performing procedures.

In my view, efficiency was not about getting all of us home earlier in the day, but rather a philosophy that efficient care is the hallmark of medical practices that provide excellent care. I rarely have seen inefficient care result in good medical care. As Norman Shumway, a renowned Stanford heart surgeon, was fond of saying, "We can do it badly or we can do it slowly, but let's not do it badly and slowly." I took that to heart.

Not everyone on staff was excited to adopt these changes. I drove the nurse manager, Carol Anderson, quite crazy with my approach. She had been with the program for many years and closely adhered to the protocols established before my arrival—from the way we immunosuppressed the patients and treated infections to how long we required out-of-town patients to live in our area (up to a year). These protocols went into the trash. Carol probably spent her first few months with me wishing she could send me back to Colorado.

The surgical team noticed the number of changes I was making as well. The person who recruited me to Stanford, senior surgeon Andrew Stevens, was a congenial guy from the Florida Panhandle and, as we say in the South, as smooth as a gin and tonic at sunset. He was one of my strongest advocates until he began to hear complaints from my surgical colleagues that I was making too many waves. Only then did he begin to question my methods. Andrew was never quick to get angry, but after hearing from one of the senior surgeons that I'd said the program was "stuck in the Stone Age," he confronted me in the ICU. Looking me right in the eye, he said, "You ought to temper your comments. We had a pretty good program long before you got here."

Which wasn't exactly true, given the recent number of transplants performed and the poor outcomes. I wasn't being asked to come to Stanford because things were going well. Quite the contrary. The leaders there wanted something different, a thriving program that reflected the excellence of the institution. And that's what I wanted as well.

Nonetheless, I felt bad in that moment, because Andrew had been in my corner, and I respected him and wanted to do right by him. Still, it was more important to me to do right by my patients, so when aspects of the program struck me as suboptimal, I was not going to just let things go to keep the peace. As our chief medical officer put it, "You're giving the program a good hard shake." I couldn't tell if he said it with admiration or disdain. It didn't really matter to me. I felt as though I was on a quest, a righteous crusade, and anyone standing in the way was either inadequately committed or didn't get it.

My motives to create the best transplant program in the world were twofold: First, to save lives. Second, to show my colleagues around the world that I could create excellence.

That's when things would get complicated.

Two

Although I had worked hard most of my medical career, I cranked it up a few notches during my first year at Stanford. There was so much to do to elevate the program to what I thought it could be, and I wanted it all to happen right away. Patience was not a strength of mine, and the new program was a perfect outlet for my restless energy. My days started early, with a 4:00 a.m. wake-up without an alarm clock and 5:00 a.m. boot camp classes at the gym, followed by bike rides up one of the mountains west of Stanford. These grueling morning rituals got me amped up for my long days at work.

The rest of a typical day looked like this: At the hospital by 7:00 a.m. to check on what had happened with the patients overnight, go on hospital rounds with the team at 8:00 a.m., see outpatients in the clinic from 9:00 a.m. to noon, a quick lunch, and then meet with hospital administrators to discuss program finances and business development, and meet with family members whose loved ones were in the hospital. Throughout the day and night, I fielded calls from the organ procurement organization (OPO) that was responsible for offering our team donor lungs when they became available.

Despite the tragedy inherent with becoming an organ donor, taking a call about a lung donor was one of my favorite parts of being a transplant doctor. When the cell phone would ring, I would recognize the number of the OPO and get an adrenaline rush. It was game time.

The procurement process is a complex one. The doctor who identifies a brain-dead donor is usually, but not always, some distance from our hospital. The hospital obtains consent from the patient's family, which, sadly, is the outcome only about half the number of times families are approached. There are arrangements made to bring the deceased patient to the operating room, where as many as eight organs might be removed to send to various facilities. In our case, our team might use one or more of these organs, but there were often multiple transplant teams from various locations sometimes—literally elbowing in to get to the deceased donor, remove a particular organ, and fly (or drive) back to where the transplant would occur.

The process is often disorderly and anachronistic, badly in need of rethinking, but like many aspects of transplant medicine, or medicine in general, motivated by profit motive and control. In my view, the procurement process should be centralized—we should set up a more cost-effective system. Instead of each transplant hospital flying someone to a donor hospital (at great expense in terms of physician time and money) to obtain the organs, they could be procured by experts in this specialized area of transplantation. The organs could be sent to the transplant hospitals, preferably using a system that keeps organs "alive" during the transportation. This sure seems more efficient than how we are doing it now.

Of all the dinnertime interruptions, calls about organ donors were the most frequent. I cared deeply about all the patients on our waiting list and viewed it as a personal failure if we could not get someone transplanted. For many who work in transplant, having a patient die on the waiting list is a sad but inevitable reality. To me, it was absolutely unacceptable.

Donor lungs come in varying degrees of quality. The top programs distinguish themselves by using lungs of seemingly lesser quality while still achieving successful outcomes. For example, we have learned over the years that older donors, defined as more than sixty years of age, can work well if all else is fine with these older lungs. Or if the donor had smoked cigarettes, these lungs are okay if there are no signs of emphysema. If there are signs of mild, clinically insignificant infections in the airways of the donor's lungs, they can be used, since we give powerful antibiotics to the lung recipient after transplant. Studies have shown, including one I published early in my career, these patients would not develop pneumonia, and their lungs would continue to do well.

One of my initial qualms with Stanford was that I felt the program was too selective about which donor lungs to accept for transplant. If a program is too conservative in their selection of donor lungs, too many patients die on the waiting list. There is then a scarcity of viable lungs and a surplus of patients who need them. Conversely, if a program is too aggressive, sometimes the new lungs won't work. There is a fine line between being too conservative and too aggressive, and straying too far in either direction leads to dead patients.

I was confident in my ability to select good donor lungs, which is an understatement if you ask the people with whom I worked. I had been taking donor calls for years prior to coming to Stanford, including long stretches of doing so every night—not recommended if you're interested in remaining sane. I learned from some of the best surgeons and transplant pulmonologists in the field about who is and who is not a suitable donor. Of everyone at Stanford, I had the most experience in selecting donors, so I took over that process entirely.

Since I'm not a surgeon, my part in the process was determining whether a set of lungs was acceptable for one of our patients. Someone on the other end of the phone would read off to me clinical parameters of the brain-dead donor, sometimes when I was at a dinner party or reading at night to my kids—the oxygenation level, the chest X-ray findings, the cause of death, how much they smoked, if they had pneumonia. I would give the thumbs-up or -down. My mental posture when deciding to accept or reject lungs was aggressive but careful. I knew that if I were overly conservative and could never pull the trigger, turning down lung after lung because it wasn't perfect, our patients would die waiting on the list, silently screaming to me, *Pull the trigger, asshole. I'm dying over here.*

Conversely if my decisions were reckless, and I took poor-quality lungs that came my way, the patient would die after implantation because the lungs wouldn't function. A decent amount of responsibility, which I relished but also made me a little crazy, because I made the error, at times, of trusting only my own judgment. I wanted to make the decision alone, just me and my waiting list. Not exactly conducive to a team sport like transplant.

Throughout the day, wherever I was—the hospital, home, at my kid's school play—I would check and recheck the waiting list, a nervous tic and frequent reminder of my life-and-death responsibility. I even felt superstitious at times. *If I touch the list, it might make the OPO call me with the most tremendous set of lungs.*

My style was a means to an end, and it was effective at getting the most people transplanted. We saved lives. The program's reputation swelled. As our volume increased and our patients continued to do well, I used our success to justify the changes I had implemented in our treatment protocols and program culture.

This success was not lost on higher-ups at the hospital, including those counting the money our program was bringing in. I perceived a causal link between my arrival and our program's improvement. This link was like an adrenaline shot to my ego, which had gotten me this far. It wasn't always pretty, but I didn't change my approach as it was working, after all.

Three

I walked into my office during my first year at Stanford, feeling tired and stiff from my morning bike ride. I changed out of my cycling clothes into green scrubs and then stretched a bit. I plopped down on the couch in my office, placed the stack of charts on the floor in front of me, and picked the first one off the top. Carol, our nurse in charge, had placed a yellow sticky note on the front of the chart that read, "Cancer. Turn down?"

In general, cancer patients are risky as transplant candidates. First, if the cancer has spread outside the chest, replacing the lungs will not be enough to cure the metastatic disease. Second, because of the powerful role of the immune system in beating back cancer mutations, the immunosuppressive drugs used after transplant to prevent rejection can allow cancers (even those confined to the chest) to spread quickly.

I scanned through the patient details: Dexter. Age thirty-six. From Nashville. Athletic, healthy. Former college football player. There was also a letter addressed to me from the patient, which wasn't typical.

Dear Dr. Weill,

My name is Dexter. I am 36 years old and I have a type of lung cancer called bronchoalveolar carcinoma (BAC). I never smoked a day in my life. I have asked several transplant programs if they would consider me for transplant. They all said they don't do transplants in patients with any type of cancer.

I found an article you wrote from Birmingham about your success transplanting people with BAC. I would like to be considered for a transplant at your program. I have two small children and have a lot to live for.

Sincerely,
Dexter

I read the letter again, pursing my lips. This guy was just a bit younger than I, also with two young children. He didn't smoke. He'd just had bad luck. Dexter's situation reminded me of Brian, my patient in Dallas who had developmental delay, causing some programs to turn him down for a transplant.

I closed the chart and attached another sticky note to the front to Carol: "To see me. Full evaluation."

A few weeks later, I saw Dexter in the clinic. He'd flown in alone from Nashville the night before. Many of our patients came from far away, adding travel burdens to the stress of an upcoming transplant operation.

We shook hands when I walked into the room, and I asked him to sit down. Built like the fullback he'd been in college, he barely fit into the chair.

Dexter didn't look sick, except for his eyes; they revealed sadness, uncertainty, worry. The moment I walked through the door he started to read me as well, looking for clues as to whether I would help him or be just another disappointment.

I started in with some small talk to put him at ease. "Please don't tell me you're a Titans fan."

He didn't crack a smile. "Yeah, always have been."

"Well, I'm a big Saints fan, so I'll need to get past that and try to like you anyway." I smiled at him, and he looked back at me blankly. He wasn't here to talk about football. He was here to see if I could help save his life. Small talk would need to wait.

After getting details of his medical history, I moved on.

"So, Dexter, as you know, most programs don't transplant people with lung cancer," I started.

"I already know that. But you did and had good outcomes in Birmingham." He got a folder out of his shoulder bag and placed it on the office desk. "The patients did fine," he reminded me. "Even better than the other patients you transplanted." He pulled the articles out of the folder and handed them to me. I set them down on the desk without looking at them.

"Yes, true enough, but we've never done that here at Stanford," I said. I was being frank; before my arrival the program had never transplanted a patient with any lung cancer, let alone the kind of lung cancer he had. "And I don't know if the surgical team—"

"You're director of the program, right?" He was calling me out.

"Yes," I said a bit defensively, "but it's a democracy, Dexter."

"But since you had this unique experience, don't you want to bring it to Stanford?"

If you only knew, I thought. "Yes, absolutely, I do. I'll talk about your case with the rest of the team, but I can't make any guarantees."

"I don't expect any sure thing, but you'll go to bat for me?" He looked at me, and I right back at him. I saw a man who'd been served a death sentence, who would do anything to live. My mind switched immediately toward yes—there would be no more doctor talk, no more qualifying every statement and "I'll do what I can" bullshit.

"You bet I will. I'll get it done," I said, locking onto his eyes as we shook hands.

I told him we'd be back in touch after our Friday meeting and wished him safe travels home. Then I went into our clinic conference room to find Carol, who was talking with one of the social workers about Dexter.

"What did you think?" she asked.

"Liked him. Put him on the agenda for the Friday meeting."

"What about the cancer? We've never done that here."

"Yeah, that and a lot of other things. Time to grow up." I laughed, trying to take the edge off my biting comment, but could tell it didn't really help.

"Okay," Carol said, shaking her head.

As I turned to walk out, Jennifer Walters, the transplant social worker, asked to speak with me in the hallway. Jennifer had been with the program a long time and I was still trying to figure out if she was on my side or not, whether she would roll with my changes to the program's culture.

"I did a social work evaluation on Dexter, and I have concerns," she said.

I checked my phone. I'd already made my decision and wasn't feeling open to hearing her evaluation.

"Do you want to know what they are?"

"Sure," I said while answering an email. I hoped she would keep it brief.

"Well, he seems angry."

I looked up from my phone and squinted at her. I could feel my face getting red. "You mean, he's angry because he's got a terminal illness and will be dead in a few months if we don't do anything? That he'll have to leave his wife and two small kids behind? Do you think that could be what's making him angry?" I couldn't contain the sarcasm. "Why should he be angry? The nerve of him."

"That's not what I meant. It's how he's handling it."

"He's handling it the best he can," I said, willing myself to regain composure. "Like any of us would hope to. He's fine. We'll talk about it on Friday."

Four

Two days later it was time for the weekly recipient selection meeting. I got to the room before anyone else, like I always did, enjoying the quiet.

The members of the transplant team sat down as they entered, and since I was leading the meeting today because Andrew was on a conference call, we started exactly at 7:00 a.m.

"Okay," I began. "Our only patient to discuss today is a guy named Dexter. He's a thirty-six-year-old man with bronchoalveolar carcinoma who is otherwise healthy. His cardiac evaluation was normal, and he has no evidence of any other organ dysfunction. He lives and works in Nashville and is married with two small kids. Jennifer, psychosocial evaluation?" She was sitting right behind me, and I turned around in my chair and gave her a long look.

"He's fine," she stated blandly.

I nodded at her and resumed. "Questions from anyone?" I looked around the room, hoping no one would say anything so we could approve Dexter for transplant and move on. I was eager to call him to deliver the good news. But as I thought about how I would tell Dexter, Johan Karlsson, one of the senior cardiothoracic surgeons, spoke up.

"I guess you have some experience with lung transplant in this kind of disease, David, but it's still cancer," he said. "I'm not sure that we should be doing this."

One of the more senior and well-respected surgeons in our program, Johan was straight out of central casting, if the movie required a Swedish doctor: shoulder-length blonde hair, with a few gray hairs mixed in, reading glasses perpetually on the end of his nose, an extra-starched white doctor's coat. When he spoke, people usually listened. He'd reminded me on more than one occasion that I'd been a junior in high school at the time he started doing transplants.

Emboldened by his words, a few other younger physicians and surgeons chimed in, parroting his reservations. I took it all in, nodding and listening to all the comments.

"Look," I said, "we can stay right in the box, do a few transplants every year, and have a nice little program. But there is experience out there with transplanting patients who have this disease. The patients we transplanted in Birmingham with BAC did well. What's the point of having experience if you don't use it?" The room once again fell silent as the team considered what I'd said.

After a few moments, Johan spoke up again. "I understand you want to help this man, but maybe we should get an oncology opinion."

"We can do that, but I don't think they will be much help," I said. "You're looking at the person with the most experience with BAC in the context of lung transplant."

"That may be, but let's get oncology involved."

And with that he got up and the discussion about Dexter abruptly ended. The team filed out of the room, no doubt relieved that the meeting was over and a fight hadn't broken out.

As I was gathering my things and thinking about how to change my colleagues' minds, Andrew Stevens asked me to talk to him in his office, which was just a few doors down from the conference room.

He sat down and put his feet up on the coffee table. "Go slow, David." he counseled, "these guys will come around. Just give 'em time. You're pushing all of us out of our comfort zone—and that's good, it's why I wanted you to come here. But remember, change is hard."

"Yeah, hard for all of us. But I'll keep at it. I'll wear 'em down."

Andrew smiled. His leadership skills far exceeded my own. His demeanor and language were always diplomatic, mine less so. "We want you here and you're going to do great things. Everyone is excited by the changes you're making. Just be patient."

"That's not exactly my strong suit. And I believe you, but it doesn't look like I have the confidence of people in that room. Looks like it's me against them."

"It's not. It just feels that way." Andrew got up and walked me to his office door. "Just keep working on it."

I nodded and left. *I will. What choice do I have?*

Five

When I arrived at the hospital for rounds, the team was waiting for me in the room of our first patient. I liked to round quickly: get in, decide what to do, and move on, everything very businesslike. This became especially important as our team grew in size. Generally, I looked at the patients' medical records in my office beforehand, so I knew the day's plan for all of our inpatients before arriving at their room. As always, efficiency was key.

The first patient that day was Emily.

"Good morning, everyone," I said, quickly scanning the group. "What's up with Emily?" I knew the answer to my own question but waited for one of the nurses to summarize her case.

"Emily is thirty-two years old with cystic fibrosis. Seven years out from her first transplant and on the wait list three months for her second transplant. Her vital signs were—"

I turned to walk into Emily's room, cutting the nurse off mid-sentence. What else was there to know?

Emily had done well after her first transplant; she'd had two kids and led an active life until a few months prior, when she'd developed chronic rejection of her transplanted lungs. Chronic rejection afflicts many transplant patients, causing loss of lung function that leaves them miserable and gasping for air, similar to how they felt pre-transplant. I hated this complication—it snatched away everything the patients, and the team, had fought so hard for. Before the transplant, we warned patients that this could happen at any time, and they all feared it at the first sign of any illness, even a mild cold. Psychologically, it was a nightmare—a recurring one.

I opened the door and the stench of putrid, infected sputum hit me right away, wafting out the door and into the hallway.

"Hey, Emily, what's up?" I asked. She was sitting bolt upright in bed while her husband performed chest percussion on her—a technique in which the percussor beats the patient on the back and chest to physically dislodge secretions from the lungs.

"Not much, trying to breathe." On cue, she coughed up an outpouring of green phlegm into a Styrofoam cup. The cup was already nearly full of mucus from a long night of coughing.

"Sorry, Doc," she apologized needlessly. "Lovely."

"No need to be sorry. I love lung biscuits in the morning. Haven't even had breakfast yet." My team standing in the room smiled, trying to hide any hints of revulsion. They were used to me joking this way with patients. "Keep it up. Better out than in. Hock that shit up."

She smiled a little and looked up at me, visibly short of breath. Emily was a pretty blond woman, very thin, like most cystic fibrosis patients—the disease prevents patients from absorbing food well. Her husband looked tired and disheveled; his hair stood straight up, his face was unshaven and gray, and his eyes were bloodshot. It wasn't his first time staying up all night with her, calming her during coughing fits.

Emily's husband seemed convinced she was in trouble, and he was right. But waiting for a transplant is as much a mental test as a physical one, and my strategy had always been not to let an ounce of negativity creep into a patient's head. The best way to do this was to appear certain and upbeat, even when I wasn't feeling that way.

"You're hanging in there nicely, Emily. You look really strong to me," I lied. "We're going to get some lungs for you very soon." She nodded and lay back in her bed. I wasn't sure if she believed me. Her chest rose and fell through her hospital gown as she worked to grab air using whatever muscles could help—neck, chest, shoulders.

"I hope so," she said. "Not sure how much longer I can hang on." She was breathing too fast, which was not a good sign.

I shot a quick glance at her husband, who visibly shrank at the thought of losing her. He grabbed her hand and wrapped his other arm around her shoulders. "No, Emily. You can do this. You did it once before, you can do it again."

She took another deep breath. "Oh yeah," she said weakly. "I'm just a regular stud." *Good—sarcasm intact. I took that as a sign.*

"That's just what I was thinking, Emily," I said, taking advantage of the moment. "I need you to get well and get out on the bike with me."

"I think you'd beat me at this point."

"Maybe, but not for long. You're a lot younger than me. We're going to get you new breathing machines and you'll be back at it, working out and chasing those kids of yours."

Her blue eyes welled up with tears. "I know," she said, still looking unconvinced.

"Alright, I'll check back on you later. Don't run off, in case we find some lungs for you."

"Don't worry, I'll be here."

I left the room, walked back into the hallway, and closed the door behind me. "She doesn't have long," I said to the team outside the room.

Right then, Emily's husband walked out of the room. "Dr. Weill, can I talk to you?" he asked. Thankfully, he hadn't heard what I'd said to the team about his wife's prognosis.

Turning to the team, I said, "I'll catch up with y'all in the ICU." As they walked away, I studied his face, which was a light gray in color and showed significant distress. He got right to the point.

"Is she going to make it to the transplant?"

"Yeah, I think so," I said, sounding less certain with him than I had with Emily. As unfailingly sunny as I tried to be with patients waiting for transplants, I tended to be more realistic with their families. "We've been busy lately with lots of donor lungs being offered, so we should be able to find her something." *Should*—a parsing of words, a hedge.

"But what if you don't? She'll die, right?" he asked.

I wanted to say, *"What do you think? That's why I can't sleep at night and why I jump three feet in the air whenever my phone rings at two a.m."* Instead, I reassured him.

"That won't happen. We'll find something for her." I took the easy way out. I didn't want to admit to him, or to myself, that we might not get it done, that we might fail. So I said we'd get it done, something I felt that he needed to believe.

Some color returned to his face. "Thanks, Doc." He grabbed my arm. "I needed to hear that."

I needed to believe that myself, every day, for every patient. Our interests were aligned in our mutual need for reassurance, strength, and at times mutual self-deception about what was ahead. Patients' families wanted the transplant to happen to save their loved one's life, and I desperately needed to make it happen for them, despite whatever consequences that obsession held for me.

I pulled my arm back a bit faster than I should have. "Okay," I said, "I'll keep you posted." Then I walked off, thinking about which patient I needed to see next.

After I finished seeing patients, I went back to my office and lay down on the couch. My sleep had been choppy the night before, my thoughts stuck on Emily's situation. A few deep breaths on the sofa helped me relax. For the first time I could remember, I said a short prayer—asking God to help this courageous woman and help me to help her. The prayer was clunky but from the heart—I didn't really know how to pray, so I started "Dear God…" and went from there. Anything that might help.

Six

The next morning, on a cold gray Northern California day, I went back to see Emily. Earlier, at three o'clock that morning, one of the overnight on-call physicians had called to tell me that she was deteriorating rapidly, and to ask if I wanted her transferred to the ICU. I said no. Emily was adamant that she wanted a transplant or nothing. No mechanical ventilator, no heroic efforts to save her.

I walked into her room alone, without the team, expecting a dire scene. Emily's husband looked even worse than the day before: sleep-deprived, despondent, restless. Emily, her lips purple from lack of oxygen, looked like she was near the end. She had a mask on, providing supplemental oxygen to lungs that no longer worked—the oxygen traveling down a road to nowhere.

She couldn't even sit upright to try to breathe better. She was done. I looked across the room. On the couch were two little girls I hadn't noticed. Sitting quietly, they each tightly held stuffed animals and stared straight at their mom, branding the traumatic image into their minds. They were young, both under ten years old. But with how sick Emily looked, they could tell their lives were about to change.

I went to Emily's bed and took her hand in mine. I leaned down next to her ear. "Are you in pain? Do you need something for it? Tell me what you need."

She said nothing but squeezed my hand weakly. I made a mental note to tell the nurse to give her some morphine, not as a pain medication but rather to alleviate the suffocating feeling patients experience when dying of respiratory failure. Next, I went to the children and got down on one knee in front of the couch.

"You may not remember what I am about to tell you, but please try to," I said. "Your mother is a very brave woman. She has fought very hard because she loves you both so much. Never forget that, no matter what."

They both looked at me and nodded. As I stood back up, the older girl said, "Thank you. I know you tried hard."

"Tell the team how much we appreciate their efforts over the last seven years," Emily's husband said, tears streaming down his face. "And you take care of yourself."

I nodded and put my hand on his shoulder, fighting back tears of my own, trying to hold off until I could be alone.

I left the room and went across the hall to a supply closet. Amid all the medical equipment, I found a step stool, sat down, and burst into tears. It had been a long time since I had cried. And looking back, it wasn't just the first time I ever cried in the hospital. After fifteen years in the field, in my mid-forties, it was the first chink in my armor.

I sat there for a few minutes, thinking about those kids, about my kids. I picked up a roll of tape from one of the boxes on the shelf and tossed it toward the ceiling, the same way I had done with my basketball as a kid, lying in bed in my room, trying not to wake my parents. *I wish I could go back to that time, when the most pressing things on my mind were basketball and the Saints.*

Jennifer, the social worker on our team, had been by to see Emily and saw me sitting in the closet as she left the room. She came in and asked if I was okay. She'd never seen me this way.

"Oh, I'm just great," I said sarcastically. I fidgeted some more with the roll of tape, starting to tear off strips of exactly equal lengths, sticking each, one by one, to the closet wall. A few moments went by as she stood there watching me. Then I got up and walked past her out of the room, muttering, "I can't stand this shit."

I had forgotten about all the other successes we'd had thus far, and there were many more of those than failures. It was as if, in that moment, when things weren't working out for the patient right in front of me, all the other patient successes were forgotten. The "saves" became part of a vague, blurry background; the ones we couldn't help stood in vivid relief, front and center, an unwelcome daily companion.

Back in my office later that same day, my to-do list beckoned—a welcome distraction. The first item: Call Dexter. I had decided to put him on the waiting list after making a cursory call to one of my oncology friends, doing the bare minimum to satisfy Johan Karlsson.

One final issue we had to overcome in Dexter's situation was getting his insurance company to authorize the transplant. If a patient does not have a disease typically amenable to transplant, like BAC, then insurance companies tend to not agree to pay for the transplant, necessitating the transplant center to explain (hopefully to a doctor at the insurance company) why a transplant might work. These conversations, in my experience, mostly go well if you can provide data to support what you are trying to do for your patient.

One problem in transplant is that the data is either lacking altogether or is sparse, which reflects the evolving nature of the field. Suffice it to say, insurance companies don't always accommodate a request for transplant because it means spending money. Conversations of this sort can turn ugly when an insurance company doesn't authorize a transplant or delays the patient in getting on a waiting list. Which can be fatal.

Fortunately, in Dexter's case, I was able to get the insurance company to pay for his transplant for an unconventional diagnosis, based mostly on a published series of BAC patients our group at UAB had transplanted.

It was midmorning in Nashville, and I caught Dexter at home.

"Hey, Dexter, it's David Weill with the Stanford transplant program. Look, I wanted to tell you, we decided to put you on our waiting list. We're going to get you a transplant."

There was silence on the other end for a few moments. Finally, he responded, "Okay. What do I do next?"

It was not exactly the jumping-up-and-down I expected and needed the morning after having said goodbye to Emily. But this was Dexter—a man of few words and seemingly even fewer emotions. Just trying to stay alive.

"Carol will be in touch soon to talk about logistics. I'm fired up. Hope you are," I said with all the enthusiasm I could muster on this sad day.

"Yep."

As we hung up, I received a text message from one of the nurses that Emily had passed away. I sat at my desk for a few moments. *What a job I have, watching a young mother die one moment and giving a young father the hope of a transplant the next. No wonder I'm crazy.* I wondered if everyone who did my job was affected the same way, if they experienced the same high from saving someone's brother or wife and the same crashing low from losing someone's mother or husband. I knew some in the field who coped in maladaptive ways: they drank too much or chased the nurses in the hospital. My way was just to go harder—at work, at the gym, on my bike. Back then, amping up the intensity was my only response to the challenges I faced.

But was it the best one?

Dexter waited for his transplant in an apartment near Stanford while his family stayed back in Nashville. The months of waiting dragged on. The average waiting time in most large programs is two weeks to three months, depending on the waiting list priority score, based on how sick someone is. I talked with him by phone every so often. When I acknowledged how difficult the wait could be, he brushed it off, saying he was "dealing with it." He passed the time by going to the gym to stay fit for the operation. A local Bay Area newspaper ran a story on him, interviewing us both—me about how patients manage the waiting period. I gave my usual answers—"It's best to stay as healthy as possible, to stay ready, to be upbeat"—but really, I didn't have a clue how patients did it. Watching patients go through the waiting isn't the same as being the patient who has to walk around on pins and needles for months or even years on end, waiting for the call.

After several months, a donor finally became available for Dexter: an excellent set of lungs, the right blood type, a perfect size match, fantastic oxygenation. When I called to tell him the good news, he said, "Fine. I'll be there soon," and hung up. I put down the phone and smiled, shaking my head. I couldn't believe this guy—stoic, businesslike, approaching his life-saving transplant like the engineer he was.

The surgery went well, and Dexter was able to leave the hospital quickly, ahead of schedule. On the day of discharge, his family came to pick him up, delighted by how things had turned out. As we stood waiting for the car at the front of the hospital, Dexter's wife cried, but he shed no tears. It was only when the car pulled up that I saw the first glimpse of emotion in him. He reached out to hug me, tentatively at first, and then more aggressively as we embraced. He held me for longer and tighter than I expected.

"Thanks, Dr. Weill," he said. "Everything went okay." He sounded surprised that it had all actually happened. He paused and smiled. "I'm okay." He stood back, took a huge, deep breath, and wiped away a few tears.

I put my hands on both sides of his face. "More than okay, Dexter. You crushed it."

"Thanks for taking a chance on me." He put out his hand. I grabbed it, then brought him in for another hug.

I thought back to our first conversation at Stanford, when he'd asked me to go out on a limb for him. Standing there with him now, I felt hopeful that the success of his transplant would pave the way for Stanford to do more "out of the box" transplants, for it to adopt a new program culture emphasizing innovation and consistent excellence. We did, in fact, go on to do some tough transplants in some really sick patients. The more success we had, however, the less tolerant I became of failure, in my colleagues or in myself.

Seven

Several months after Dexter's transplant, in the fall of 2009, I had a difficult conversation in clinic with Amanda, a twenty-five-year-old cystic fibrosis patient whom we had transplanted two years prior. After her transplant she had done quite well, but then her lungs began to fail, and we diagnosed her with chronic rejection. We tried every treatment option, but as in most cases of chronic rejection, nothing improved her condition. She was in clinic that day to discuss her next steps.

Amanda came with her mom, whom I had come to know well. The two were close, and they'd taken advantage of the new life Amanda's transplant had provided. Amanda had sent me pictures of them on the beach in Maui, on a ski run at Tahoe, and under the Eiffel Tower.

My mood was somber for this clinic visit. I sat down while mother and daughter waited for me to begin. Amanda's eyes were red and puffy from crying, and her hands clutched a box of tissues. She removed her oxygen cannula to blow her nose. The fact that she even had to use oxygen again broke my heart; she was right back to where she was when we first met, before her transplant. I rolled my chair toward her and patted her knee.

"Amanda, we've tried everything we know to try, and it doesn't look like things are getting any better," I said. "I think it's time to consider a second transplant."

Her mother started crying silently as they both nodded their heads. They had known this was coming, but to hear me actually say the words must have been devastating.

To decline like this, to return to the pre-transplant state, is the cruelest joke of our field; patients get to taste what life can be, then the plate is yanked away. I hated chronic rejection. It had robbed too many patients of their lives. It was a formidable foe, the grim reaper of lung transplant.

Amanda collected herself for a moment and then said, "I'm game. Tell me what I need to do."

"You've been through it before, so you know the drill. We'll run a few tests just to make sure everything besides your lungs is in good working order. Shouldn't be too much."

Amanda shrugged her shoulders and nodded. She had been sick since she was five—a few more tests didn't concern her.

"Okay, I'll get the ball rolling," I said. "What questions do you have?"

They were both silent for a few moments. Then, Amanda's mother asked, barely louder than a whisper, "Do you think…" She stopped to wipe a few tears away. "Do you think Amanda can make it to the transplant? Survive the wait?"

I didn't hesitate for a second. "Oh yeah," I said, nodding vigorously. "No question. We'll get her some lungs." With that I stood up, gave Amanda and her mom quick hugs, and left the room. I found one of the nurses and told her to get Amanda tested and listed as soon as possible.

A week went by, and Amanda's tests didn't reveal any surprises. I presented her case to the team in our Friday morning selection meeting, and everyone agreed she should be re-transplanted. Prior to my arrival, Stanford had not done many re-transplants, and the ones that had been done had not had very good outcomes. Soon after I started working there, we had decided to stop doing second transplants for about a year so we could review our protocols and techniques. Re-transplants present more technical difficulties, because transplanted lungs develop scar tissue that adheres to the chest wall. Getting these lungs out during the second transplant is no easy task, and patients often bleed a lot during the lung extraction, significantly adding to the morbidity, and in some cases the mortality, of the operation.

Still, re-transplantation was becoming common at other large programs across the world, and I felt like we owed it to patients to offer it—as long as we could do it well. I worked with the medical directors at the various large insurance carriers to explain our reasoning and what I thought the outcomes might be.

The insurance companies came to understand that re-transplants can work well in carefully selected candidates and, after some cajoling, agreed to authorize Amanda's second transplant and subsequently those of many other patients. A human connection with the insurance companies, in this case doctor to doctor, can impact their decisions. Usually, if a patient or even a nurse goes through the usual channels to seek authorization for a riskier procedure, the first answer is no. I chose, in this instance and many others, to pick up the phone and find a human, preferably a doctor, with whom I could form a personal connection. This time it had worked.

Amanda would be the first re-transplant patient listed at Stanford after the program's yearlong hiatus from the procedure. Now that she was listed, her wait—and ours— had begun.

Eight

About a month later, a donor became available for Amanda. It was just in time. I had seen her in clinic just a few days prior, and she was declining rapidly. The amount of supplemental oxygen she needed had shot up, and she was using the maximum amount before requiring a mechanical ventilator.

The surgeon on the call schedule that night was Donald Bowman, a pleasant guy but not very experienced with lung transplant. He was unfailingly polite, a product of a farming community in Kansas, built like a running back, with bright red hair. But like most young surgeons, he was conservative in his donor lung selection.

And one could understand why this can happen, if there is some doubt in the minds of the transplant doctors: better not to do the transplant at all than to accept a pair of donor lungs that don't work. To many in the transplant field, a death on the waiting list was one thing, not desirable certainly, but less catastrophic than a death after transplant. A post-transplant death would adversely affect program survival statistics and might prompt regulatory scrutiny. It could also diminish a surgeon's reputation.

But to me, a waiting list death or a death after transplant was a distinction without a difference—dead is dead. I know there was no difference to our patients and their families.

The problem with being too conservative in donor selection, since all of our patients were at risk of dying on the list, was that we couldn't wait for the perfect set of lungs. We had to take a risk—a calculated risk, an unblinking one, but a risk nonetheless. Risk was not something we had the option of avoiding—it was part of our business.

Waiting for another set of donor lungs to come along was essentially making a tacit bet the patient wouldn't die while we waited for something better. It was a gamble. To do transplant work, you need to accept this reality. The critical question was not whether the donor lungs were perfect, but whether they would work for one of our dying patients.

Donald called me to discuss the details of Amanda's donor, a twenty-four-year-old man who had died in car accident, but it had not adversely affected his lung function. As I explained to Donald, these lungs would be a trade up from her current ones. He didn't think so and resisted my pushing.

"I don't know, David," he said. "I know you have more experience with donors, but this one worries me."

I was at home pacing, walking fast laps around my kitchen. It was the middle of the night (when most donor calls happen), and my family was asleep, so I tried to keep my voice down. "What worries you?" I asked, whispering, enunciating each word with extra bite.

"The chest contusion," he said. This kind of "bruise" can sometimes negatively affect lung function, but is often no big deal, as in this situation. "It's a contraindication to lung donation," he said.

I was shaking my head in frustration, walking even faster now. "Only if the lungs are adversely affected. These are working great. Let's take 'em."

"I don't know. Let me ask someone else," Donald said.

Who the hell are you going to ask? I wanted to say. *I've been taking donor calls since the early 1990s. These are fine.*

"Donald, I'm making the call," I finally said. "Let's do it. I've taken lots of lungs just like these, and they've worked fine." In reality, I wasn't his boss and couldn't force him to do the transplant. But I could sure as hell try to convince him to see my point of view.

"I don't think we should do it."

The back-and-forth went on and on for several minutes. Finally, I interrupted him. "You understand that she's dying, right? That she's on our list for a reason?"

I thought back to the day in clinic when I'd reassured Amanda and her mom that we'd find her lungs.

I wasn't going back to sleep—I never could after a donor call came in. And while it always upset me to have to turn down an opportunity to transplant, this time I was furious. When I first got to Stanford, we'd all made an agreement that we would only do a transplant if both the surgeon and I agreed to go ahead. In effect, each of us had veto power. My job was to influence the decision, but ultimately I couldn't, and wouldn't, make a surgeon do a transplant he didn't feel good about.

The lungs would go elsewhere that night—maybe out of state, or possibly to a waiting patient at the UC San Francisco transplant program. At least someone would get them, albeit not one of our patients. Needing distraction, I went out to my garage office and answered emails until dawn.

I spent the next few days worrying about Amanda and stewing about my conversation with Donald. Thankfully, another donor came up for her within the week. This was rare in many parts of the country, but not in Northern California, where the donation rates were very good.

Many factors were involved in having a plentiful supply of donor organs in our area, among them a high population density—lots of people leads to lots of potential donors—and the higher education and socioeconomic status that usually is associated with higher donation rates.

Once again, Donald was the surgeon on call. He texted me that we had a donor for Amanda, and I took a few moments to gather myself before I got ready for Act Two.

I called Donald's cell, and he picked up on the first ring. "Hello, David, how are you?" he asked, a bit too enthusiastically for 2:00 a.m. I looked for something to eat as he continued with the pleasantries. "So sorry to wake you. Can I talk to you about a donor?"

Donald proceeded to tell me, in painful detail, about the donor. Eager for the punch line, I took control of the conversation, firing off questions about the specific aspects of the donor I was interested in. The lungs, again, sounded fine to me.

"The donor smoked cigarettes," Donald said, "and that's a contraindication to lung transplant donation."

I tried to count to ten, but only made it to three before I lost it. "Sure, Donald, if he smoked every day of his life! He smoked a few cigarettes in high school. Who didn't?"

"I still don't think we should take the lungs, David."

I walked to the front door of our house and quietly closed it behind me, trying not to disturb Jackie and the kids. Standing in front of my house in my robe, my entire body was shaking with rage. "Look, no disrespect, but it doesn't look like you can pull the trigger. It's time to do this transplant. This girl is going to die. Meaning dead. Meaning not coming back. Let's do what we're paid to do."

"Seems risky, David."

Now I was on the move in our cul-de-sac, walking in the middle of the street, arms flailing, my billowing dark-green robe like a tent about to blow off a mountaintop.

"You know what's risky, Donald?" I paused for full effect, took the phone away from my ear, and held the speaker up to my mouth. "Not doing the fucking transplant." I was now leaning toward the phone, bent at the waist. "Not giving the girl a chance. Now take these fucking lungs, and let's get it done."

"I don't understand why you need to use that language."

"Look, I'll talk to my shrink about it. In the meantime, can we possibly get a transplant done?"

No response from his end. He was thinking, and I was walking down the street, looking into the windows of my neighbors' houses, hoping no one was awake and watching me.

"Okay, David, I guess it will be okay."

I hung up, satisfied that Amanda was going to get the transplant, but sorry that I'd had to be such a prick to get it done. I never wanted to be so rude, but it seemed to be the only way to advocate for my patient.

Here is how I justified my behavior: I lacked patience and tact when lives were on the line. I was on a mission—

what I considered a righteous, life-saving mission—that could appear to an outside observer to be a sort of transplant mania. My need to continue on this path was more important than anything else, including any work relationship. I am sure Donald wanted the same thing—he was just a young guy trying to do the right thing that night. But we had different approaches. No patients were not going to die on my watch. And there would be no negotiation.

Nine

I was waiting in my Stanford office for the call that Amanda was out of surgery. The surgical team was supposed to have finished early that morning, but at 3:00 p.m., there was still no word. This is never a good thing. Often, a longer time in the operating room means complications have developed, like uncontrollable bleeding or difficulty extracting the old lungs.

I looked for anything to take my mind off the worst-case scenario—wiping my computer keyboard with alcohol swabs, throwing away papers from my desk, rearranging the stacks of clean dress shirts I kept in my office. Next, I lay down on the couch with my basketball, shooting it toward the ceiling, the simple ritual I used to calm myself. As I waited, my mind kept jumping to consider all the scenarios that could be going on in the operating room.

Finally, an hour later, the ICU doctor, Helen Stewart, texted me that Amanda was in the ICU. I hurried down the one flight of stairs, unsure what to expect and bracing myself for the worst. On my way, I saw Amanda's mom and stopped to tell her I would come talk to her once I had assessed the situation. I didn't want to seem worried, so I purposely slowed my pace. The last thing a patient's family needs to see is their loved one's doctor running frantically to the ICU.

I passed through the automatic double doors. Normally, as soon as these doors open, a low roar can be heard—doctors and nurses talking and moving hurriedly, the ICU's heightened sense of urgency audible. Today it was quiet.

I could tell which room was Amanda's: the one with a big crowd. My heart sank. After a transplant that goes well, the crowd thins out quickly.

I found Helen in the midst of the crowd. She was an earnest, careful physician who led the ICU team in charge of Amanda's care. She emerged from the crowd when she saw me, a worried look on her face, and began to fill me in.

"Amanda just got out and has had a rough time," she said. "Apparently the team had trouble getting the old lungs out, so the donor lungs sat in the ice chest in the OR for two hours."

I closed my eyes for a moment. Disaster.

The timing of a transplant is critical, carefully choreographed to ensure that the old lungs come out before the donor lungs even arrive. Once the new lungs are removed from the donor's body, they must be implanted into the recipient as quickly as possible. The longer they are outside a body, the less likely the transplant will be a success.

Amanda's new lungs had been out of her donor's body for nine hours, at least twice as long as ideal. Her old lungs were so diseased, they were essentially stuck to her chest wall by all the scar tissue. This is not uncommon in cystic fibrosis patients with their infected, purulent lungs, especially in those receiving a second transplant.

In Amanda's case, by the time the surgeons had meticulously dissected the old lungs free, the new lungs in the ice bucket were "growing hair," as one of my mentors liked to say. The chances they would work were small.

"She is not oxygenating well, despite maximum ventilator settings," Helen said, "and she's bleeding some."

This was the understatement of the year. I looked over at Amanda. The white blankets covering her were now mostly red, the blood soaking through them and dripping onto the floor.

"Okay. Thanks." I took a deep breath and walked up to her bed and pulled back her blanket. The nurse asked me if I wanted some gloves. I heard her but didn't answer.

I didn't intend to be rude, but this was the climactic moment of my worst nightmare. A horror show was unfolding before my eyes, and there was nothing I could do. Her chest had been left open by the surgical team because the new lungs were so swollen that they didn't fit inside her chest. The open chest allowed more space for the edematous lungs that ideally would shrink back down to normal size after a day or two.

Blood pooled in her open chest cavity and seeped down her legs. I looked at her transplanted lungs—angry, red, and bloated like two big, wet sponges. I knew right away that these weren't going to work. Not now, and likely not ever.

The bedside monitor showed the telltale signs of postoperative distress: low blood pressure and poor oxygenation. I had seen enough. I backed away from the bed and walked into the hallway, where Helen was talking to Donald, who had performed the surgery.

Amanda needed a miracle to survive, and I calmly stated the obvious. "Looks like things didn't go well. I'll go talk to her mother."

In the waiting room, Amanda's mother sat with a man I'd never seen. They stood up as I came in, and the man introduced himself as Amanda's father. We sat down and I gave them a quick summary: Amanda's operation had been difficult; we were doing the best we could. Essentially, we'd expected things to be tough, and that's what had come to pass.

Amanda's mother cried as I talked. Her father's eyes never lost contact with mine. When I was done explaining the situation, I gave her mom a hug and put my hand on her dad's shoulder. "I'll come back and give you an update in a little while," I promised.

Walking away from the conversation, it finally sank in that—even with the ICU team doing everything in their power to keep Amanda alive—she probably would not make it. Her fate had been sealed by an unfortunate sequence of events: the lungs had simply been in the ice chest too long, deprived of the much-needed blood flow and ventilation that keeps them "alive." A mentor used to say that, in transplant, "Bad starts lead to bad finishes." And this transplant had had a very bad start.

Back in my office, I stretched out again on the couch. *What more can we do for Amanda? List her again and try to do another transplant?* Her life expectancy at this point was a few hours. There was no chance we would find another set of donor lungs in that time frame. She was losing too much blood to do much of anything except transfuse her and pray.

She was already receiving transfusions, so much so the hospital blood bank was rapidly running out of stock.

I felt helpless, bitter that Amanda's circumstances were beyond my ability to fix. But saying a prayer was something I could do, so I did. My need for divine intervention on Amanda's behalf was urgent, even though at that point, religion did not yet play a large role in my life.

As I fumbled for the right words, I was interrupted by a text from Helen, asking me to come back to the ICU right away. Amanda was going downhill fast.

The crowd outside Amanda's room was gone. Helen was standing in the hall.

"She's gotten twenty units of blood, David," she said. "We still can't keep her blood pressure up, and we can't get her to oxygenate at all. She hasn't made any urine, so her kidneys are shutting down. And her liver is starting to take a hit, based on her liver function studies."

"Besides that, everything is going great," I said. I didn't know what else to say. We were both at a loss.

"Yeah, she's up against it. What do you want to do?" she asked.

I rocked back and forth from heel to toe and circled my neck around—nervous habits. I then did a deep knee bend and stayed in a squat. Helen stared at me, puzzled.

I stood back up. "Let's stop," I said. "We have to let her go."

"I think that's the right thing to do. You sure you're okay with that?"

"No. But it's what we need to do." I forced a half smile. "I'll go talk with the family. Thanks for your efforts, Helen."

Amanda's parents were sitting in the empty waiting room, her father's arm around her mother, comforting her as she cried. Her father looked up at me as I walked up, but her mother didn't, as if not engaging with me would keep the tragedy from being real.

I pulled up a chair across from them and sat for a few minutes. Except for soft sobs, the room was silent. Chairs were scattered about, and empty fast-food bags littered the floor. The smell of greasy food was overpowering.

In situations like these, in which family members know what I am going to say, I find it's best to just get the words out—to rip the Band-Aid off.

"Amanda is not going to make it," I said. "We've tried everything, and she hasn't responded. We need to stop her from suffering."

Earlier in my career, I would have asked the family if they wanted to stop all aggressive care and let their loved one pass on. But as end-of-life discussions became more commonplace for me, I came to understand one of the hardest things for families is to make the proactive decision to end their loved one's life.

I had begun to tell families what we would be doing, what we should be doing. This approach transferred the decision-making burden from them to me. While somewhat paternalistic, this method relieves families of a huge burden. It enables them to view the process as a doctor's mercy in helping to end their loved one's suffering.

Amanda's mother didn't look up. Her father spoke. "We know you did everything you could, Doctor. We appreciate it. And we know Amanda fought to stay alive, but we don't want her to suffer. She's done that all her life, except for a few years after her first transplant. The years you gave her."

I swallowed hard. *Years that I gave her?*

I was humbled that he saw it that way, but looking back now, I don't believe that's what happened. Patients fight for their lives and are saved by a gift from their donor, by their determination, and by help from above—for those who believe in this sort of intervention. I help facilitate the gift by performing my clinical duties, but for the longest time I thought that my medical interventions were not only the key determinant of a patient's survival, I thought they were the only one.

Back then, I considered Amanda's death a personal and an institutional failure. It's only today, twenty-five years into my transplant career, that I see the arrogance of that mind-set. Just as I didn't *save* hundreds of lives with my extraordinary talent, I didn't *kill* all the patients who died either. I didn't have the wisdom to see that then.

I was waging a personal war against death, and I thought I should be able to win each and every battle. This way of thinking was a misunderstanding of my place in the world and of my role in the transplant process, but I felt at the time that it helped me be the best transplant doctor I could be. I found that same arrogance, that belief in my ability to control outcomes, had an upside: it served to instill confidence in the patients who put their lives in my hands. But death wasn't as simple as a referendum on my job performance.

Back in the waiting room, I gave Amanda's mother one last hug and left.

Amanda's father followed me down the hall. I heard a voice behind me, "Dr. Weill?"

I turned around and was face-to-face with him. "Are you okay?" he asked. *He's in the process of losing his daughter—his only child—and he's asking me if I'm okay?*

I nodded and shrugged my shoulders, as if to say, "Sure. I'm fine." But my eyes filled with tears, giving me away. I tried to stop myself. *Think about what he's going through, David, not what you're going through.* I found a few words.

"There's nothing like losing a child." I kicked the gleaming hospital floor with the heel of my shoe, trying to knock the shine right off it. "I've got two daughters of my own," I said. Then two fathers looked at each other, tears spilling from both of our eyes. Nothing else to say, no way to improve on the silence we shared.

Back in my office, I rubbed my eyes and sat on the couch, staring straight ahead, looking at a picture on the wall of me with my first transplant patient from the mid-'90s, my beaming smile revealed an exhilaration that seemed so very far removed from how I felt now. I sat there crying, not only because I would miss Amanda's smiling face in our clinic, but because the therapy I provided, the treatment I tried so hard to deliver, was by its very nature imperfect—and imperfect in wholly unpredictable ways. Intellectually, I understood that. Emotionally, I couldn't accept it.

Every transplant program, whether in our hospital or someplace else, has an ever-present companion: death. Some days your patients dodge it, and maybe even weeks go by and you stop thinking about it for a while. But you can be under no illusion—death will circle back, a constant shadow lurking around the next corner.

Watching people die, people to whom I had grown attached—like Emily, like Amanda, like others before them—forced me to face the fact that there were limitations to what I could do. Somehow, that was something I had never considered before that moment.

I had entered the field years ago, enticed by the possibility of delivering great successes. But the exhilaration of the saves turned out to be no consolation for the losses. Transplantation had become utterly bad for my psyche, though the chance to compete with death, to cheat it, to outsmart it, was still intoxicating. But the quest for perfection, which had been so alluring when I was a younger doctor, began to seem frivolous as I matured.

In the immediate aftermath of losing Amanda, I had not yet evolved this perspective on my limited amount of control. These observations were simply not yet part of my lexicon. Instead, I dug in harder, doubling down in my pursuit of some kind of transplant nirvana.

Ten

The day after Amanda's death the transplant team met in the ICU to see our newly transplanted patients. In general, the death of a patient puts the team in a funk for a few days, and today was no exception.

Part of my coping strategy was to limit discussion of Amanda during rounds. When one of the nurses brought her up the next morning, I told the team we would fully assess what had happened in a mortality conference in two weeks' time, as we did for any patient who had died under our care. This would give us all some perspective on what we had done well and what we could improve.

"Okay, which patient is first?" I asked. The nurses filled me in on two patients who had been transplanted in the previous week; they had both done well and were ready to leave the ICU. The first, Erin, a forty-year-old woman with cystic fibrosis, had been very nervous about her transplant. Because of her ambivalence, she had put off being listed until she couldn't wait any longer. In the weeks before transplant, she required the maximum amount of oxygen we could provide. Eventually, she transitioned to mechanical ventilation and required full blood pressure support, which she received for three days before we found donor lungs for her. When the surgeons removed her old lungs, they looked like blackened, decaying bags. Miraculously, she'd made it to transplant and was now having a smooth recovery.

In her room, I found her eating breakfast in a chair by her bed. A brief scan of the room showed 100 percent oxygen saturation on her bedside monitor and minimal bleeding in the chest tubes. She was detached from the oxygen tank that for years had been her leash, her lifeline. *All good. Thank God*, I thought, in light of the previous day's carnage.

When I expressed how happy I was with her progress, she reached out and took my right hand in hers. Her hands were warm—a startling difference from how they had felt pre-transplant, when they were like the cold hands of the dying. When I gently tried to pull my hands away, she grabbed me even tighter. I let her hold them.

"I feel great," she said. "I didn't think it was going to go this well."

"Well, it doesn't always." *Amanda.* "Thanks for making our job so easy." The nurse at the bedside smiled as she fiddled with the bags of medications at on the IV pole.

"I want to thank the whole team. You guys have been great."

"Well, you did the hard part," I said. "We'll be back to see you later."

The ten-person team trailed behind me as I walked out of the room. We were all thankful to have an uncomplicated transplant to discuss that morning.

The next patient we visited was Randall, a fifty-five-year-old man with pulmonary fibrosis, who was also doing well. This is a chronic disease that, for reasons still unknown, scars the lungs and renders them unable to pass oxygen into the blood. He was a busy executive in the technology industry and, just two days out of surgery, was sitting up in his bed, checking emails on his laptop. I walked up to his bedside and put my hand on his shoulder.

"How we doing this morning?"

"Pretty good, just catching up on work," he said, looking up from his computer.

"We won't keep you long. I'm just checking on things." I circled the bed, doing my routine scan of the room.

"Don't want to rush things," he said, "but when can I get out of here? I've got tons to do at work."

I laughed and turned to the team behind me, then back to him. "What do you think, you just got an appendectomy? Give us a little more time."

He was smiling now and agreed to be slightly more patient. "But as soon as possible. Okay, Doc?"

"I'm hurt. I'm beginning to think you don't like me."

"No, just don't like hospitals." He smiled.

"Well, can't blame you there." Walking out, it occurred to me that I was beginning to like them less and less myself. "Home soon." I clapped my hands like a quarterback breaking a huddle. "Soon."

We were back in the hallway and on the move again, I never stood still on rounds. Keeping the team in perpetual motion made me feel like we were accomplishing something, as if activity equaled progress. The team trailed behind me. When we took the stairs, I ran up as fast as I could, two steps at a time. Behind me, shoes clacked on the hospital floor, and I overheard idle chatter from the rest of the team about patient care matters, movies, restaurants, their weekend plans. I didn't miss a word but acted as though I wasn't listening.

When I was in a good mood—which is to say, when the patients were doing well—I would look over my shoulder and throw in a joke or some gentle ribbing. We would laugh as a group as we romped around the hospital, a band of merry healers periodically being shushed by nurses. But when things didn't go well, as in Amanda's case, the team heard nothing from me, seeing only the back of my head as I rushed away.

Eleven

N ext in the lineup that morning was Ken, age forty-three, who had been transplanted due to rapidly progressive pulmonary fibrosis. Despite the fact that two weeks had passed since his surgery, he had so far been unable to come off the mechanical ventilator and breathe on his own. It was unclear why he couldn't breathe independently.

On the X-rays his lungs appeared to be fine, leading me to suspect that he was having a problem with ventilation—the mechanics of being able to inflate and deflate his new lungs. I'd seen this before in other patients and knew it could be due to a muscular problem, a neurological problem (the brain having trouble sending the signal to breathe), or a psychological problem, like postoperative depression or anxiety. I had a hunch that Ken's new lungs were fine physically. I believed he was struggling with his will to live after two tough weeks in the ICU.

Prior to surgery, Ken had given me no reason to expect that he'd have motivational problems after transplant. When I'd met him in clinic a few months earlier, he'd been personable and mission-oriented about his transplant. "Let's just get it done," he'd said over and over that day.

I liked Ken and his wife, Dottie, who accompanied him to his first clinic visit. They were an engaging couple. She was bright and organized and had shown up with a list of questions about lung transplant. Ken interjected a few questions here and there but seemed happy to let his wife ask the tough questions while he chatted with me about sports and what I liked to do with my free time. He was close to his kids. He worked as a mechanic for a company that serviced private planes, which fascinated me. I joked that, in exchange for a transplant, he could set me up with a new Gulfstream. He replied, "Sure, if you have thirty million dollars, it's yours."

Despite the fact that my other patients were doing so well, I was in a pissy mood when I walked into Ken's ICU room after his surgery. I diagnosed my mood as "the Amanda aftershock."

"Hey, Ken, good morning. How's it going?" I asked.

He couldn't respond verbally, as he was still hooked up to the ventilator, but he shook his head to imply that he was not doing well. His wife was despondent in her seat by the bed. The two weeks she'd spent tending to Ken post-transplant had thoroughly chipped away at her façade of efficiency and control. Ken's nurse, Sandy, who had been caring for him for several days, stopped what she was doing.

"I think your lungs are fine, Ken," I said, calmly and matter-of-factly. "Focus on taking slow, deep breaths, one after another, so we can get that breathing tube out of your throat." *It's just breathing, man, simple as that,* I thought, but for post-transplant patients, sometimes breathing is anything but simple, anything but automatic. Ken started shaking his head again, and as we talked his anxiety and frustration began to increase his respiration rate.

"It's now or never," I explained, this time more forcefully. "The longer you sit here in this ICU, the worse things will get, and the more likely the transplant won't work. You want to get out of here, right? Get back to living your life? That's why you got the transplant, right?" I had done this part of the transplant pep talk before. What came next, though, was uncharted territory, an unfamiliar part of the postoperative conversation.

Ken asked for a piece of paper to write a message. Sandy handed him a clipboard and a pen, and while he wrote I checked his bedside monitor and glanced at the TV. The news was showing footage of then-Senator Barack Obama campaigning about bringing hope and change to America. I found myself thinking that if he could just bring hope and change to Ken, he'd have my full support. Ken handed me the clipboard.

"This—not working. I want to die."

I was stunned. Pursing my lips, I considered his words for a few seconds, then handed the clipboard to Sandy. She read the message before gently placing the clipboard at the foot of the bed. In less than a minute, my mentality shifted from that of a motivator, cheering my patient on to good health, to that of a disciplinarian. I was pissed off, and ready to open up a can of (old-school transplant) "whoop-ass." To do this right, I wanted to clear the room.

Dottie read the clipboard, too. I asked if she would give Ken and me some time to talk alone, but she insisted on staying. *Suit yourself*, I thought. *This isn't going to be pretty.*

Sandy stayed, too, which I wasn't thrilled with, but I forged ahead anyway.

Once it was just the four of us, I began to wind up. "First of all, you don't know how lucky you are," I started. "Do you know how many young people—younger than you—I've watched die? And not in a pretty way. People with kids and parents who desperately wanted them to live. A lot of my patients would do anything to get the chance you have." I could feel myself heating up. "You *will* not waste it. I *will* not let you."

Ken started shaking his head again, this time with more vigor, his forehead wrinkled and face contorted. I could feel Sandy and Dottie's wife's eyes drift over to Ken, then to me, then back to Ken.

"You are *not* going to waste this transplant and dishonor your donor's family by quitting just because things got hard." I turned up the volume, my words precise and clipped. "You are going to stop slugging around, start breathing, and get off this damn ventilator." My face was reddening, and I felt hot, like lava was erupting up my neck and out through my scalp. I had escalated from controlled indignation to rage.

Ken squinted at me with hatred and gestured for someone to hand him the clipboard. Without speaking, he still communicated so much. He took the pen and triple-underlined the phrase, "I want to die," then handed the clipboard back to me. I tossed it onto the bed. Sandy had turned away from the conversation and was fumbling with the IV drips and working at the bedside computer—a nurse's equivalent of finding a rock to hide under.

I leaned in closer to the bed, now hovering over Ken, inches from his face. Dottie got up from her chair and took a step toward the bed.

"Here's the deal, Ken," I said. "In *this* hospital, on *this* transplant service, no one dies until I say so." It was a line my former mentor, Marty Zamora, coined back when I was training with him. I had never said it to a patient before, but I felt this was the perfect opportunity to pull it off the shelf. "If you want to sit on the ventilator for the rest of your life, fine. Take it home with you, if you make it that far."

Sandy stopped what she was doing and stared at me.

"Enjoy yourself tonight," I continued. "But you want to know what I'm doing tonight? I'm going to go home, eat dinner with my family, and crawl into bed with my wife at the end of the night. That's what I'm going to do. You can do whatever you want, stay on the vent or try to come off. But I'm not letting you quit on this transplant and die. Suck it up."

I backed away and looked at Sandy and Dottie, both of whom were sobbing, shaking their heads in disbelief, and wiping their noses with tissues. I glanced back up at the monitor again: Ken's respiratory rate, blood pressure, and heart rate were all way up. He was agitated. I was glad—it meant I had achieved the desired therapeutic effect.

I walked out of the room, shoulders thrown back. I had used the last weapon in my arsenal to motivate Ken, and I hoped it would work. I also hoped I wouldn't get fired over it. Donor lungs are scarce, and I was angry that I'd had to be so extreme to get Ken to understand the obligation that comes with receiving them.

Sandy came out of the room and called out to me. "Dr. Weill, was that really necessary?" she asked. "Did you need to be that harsh?"

"Not now," I said, slamming my fist into the button that opens the double doors. Sandy and I had worked together long enough that she had seen me at my best before. Now she was seeing me use unconventional techniques to get the patient where he needed to go. Despite knowing that I'd had good intentions, I knew she would never be able to condone my method.

Outside the ICU, the team was waiting for me.

"How'd it go with Ken?" one of the nurses asked.

Still enraged, I said curtly, "Who's next?" We proceeded to see other patients. They knew me well enough to let it go.

Twelve

That night, the ICU nurse manager had emailed me that Sandy was upset and hinted that she might need to bring the incident to the attention of the hospital's higher-ups. I hoped to avoid that situation, if possible, so the next day, before I went back to see Ken, I stopped to talk to Sandy.

I found her outside his room, doing charting work on the computer. I walked up behind her and put my hand on her shoulder. She turned to face me and scanned different parts of my face, as though she wanted to say something but was holding back.

"Look, I'm sorry you were upset," I said before she could speak. "I don't want to say things like that to a patient, but it's my responsibility to get him home. And I'll do anything it takes, including yelling at him, to make that happen."

"I understand, David," she said, smiling. She knew my motives were pure, even if the means to the end could sometimes be crude. Plus, in this instance at least, my methods had worked. She nodded toward Ken, who gave me a thumbs-up from behind the sliding glass door that opened into his room.

"He's been breathing on his own all night long and this morning," she continued. "He looks great. I think we can take the breathing tube out."

I nodded and waited for a second, expressing nothing outwardly while inwardly celebrating. *Yes! Fucking yes! I'm one bad motherfucker*, I thought. I squeezed my right hand tightly into a barely noticeable fist pump of triumph as I watched Ken through the glass. He was sitting up in bed, engaged, and breathing like a champion.

"I'm going in to talk to him," I said.

Sandy smiled at me again and patted me softly on the back. She knew I was stoked.

I opened the door and gave a half wave to Dottie. She didn't acknowledge me and looked angry—I assumed about the previous day's ugly encounter.

"Ken, my man. Look at you!" I said, trying to make up for my extreme behavior, expressing my excitement at his progress. "Breathing on your own! Keep this up and you're going to be out of here very soon."

He smiled at me crookedly, the tube still down his throat. Sandy came to stand next to me, and Ken gestured again for the clipboard. He scribbled "Thanks," underlined it twice, and handed it to me. I looked at the clipboard for a few moments, satisfied that what I'd done the day before—although extremely rough around the edges—had worked. *This guy was going home soon*, I thought, *and that's what matters.*

I leaned over, placed my hand on top of his head, and said, "No, thank you." My eyes moistened.

This was the best feeling in the world. I'd gone out on a limb, and I'd changed the direction of Ken's life. In this case, I felt the ends did indeed justify the means.

"Sandy," I said, "let's get that tube out of his throat." Dottie covered her mouth and began to tear up.

Right then, I loved my job. How could I not?

A few days later, Ken left the hospital, breathing without oxygen. Before the transplant, and in the immediate aftermath of the surgery, he'd been on the verge of dying; now, he was going home to his family.

After seeing him off that day, one of the nurses came to my office to drop off a note from Dottie. She handed it to me and said, "From your girlfriend, Ken's wife," giving me a little wink. I thanked her, put my feet on my desk, and read the note.

> *Dear Dr. Weill,*
>
> *I just wanted to tell you how much Ken and I appreciate what you did for us. I was so angry at you for yelling at Ken. I had never seen a doctor do that but I think it changed his mind set and got him out of the hospital. It also proved to us that you really care. We can see that your job isn't easy. Keep up the good work and thanks again.*
>
> *Best,*
> *Dottie Phillips*

I reread the letter and looked out my window, then put the letter in my patient memento box. She was right—my job was not an easy one. But on this day, it was the best one. And one worth fighting to get right.

Thirteen

One chilly morning in February 2011, I found Johan Karlsson waiting outside my office door. He had never been to my office before—the unspoken protocol was for meetings to take place in the office of the more senior physician.

Somewhat shy but always polite, Johan greeted me with a nod. I gestured toward a chair, and we both sat down.

Never having been in my office before, he slowly scanned the photos on my walls: Lance Armstrong, me pretending to be Lance Armstrong while riding up a mountain in France, my wedding photo, Martin Luther King Jr., protesting in New York City. He took his time, studying each photo in detail before his eyes moved on to the next one. He was a methodical man, and this trait made him a good surgeon.

After an awkward couple of minutes, he turned his attention back to me.

"After a lot of thought, I've decided to stop operating," he said, finally. "I want to do some traveling with my wife. It's time."

This was terrible news. Although he himself wasn't doing many of the operations anymore, he was like a god looking down on the operating room, providing calming support to the young and less-experienced members of our surgical team.

"Well, that's great, Johan, but we sure are going to miss you."

He smiled and said nothing.

After he left my office, I thought about the impact his leaving would have on the program. While he was not the agent of change I felt the program needed, he was an excellent technical surgeon. Now he was on his way out, increasing the urgency among the leaders in the hospital—and me—that recruiting a new surgical leader was necessary. I figured that Johan's exit might provide the impetus to get it done, and I made a mental note to speak with Andrew Stevens about it later in the day. In the meantime, I was due at the outpatient clinic.

At the clinic I had the opportunity to see patients that were doing well, as opposed to the sicker ones who needed to be in the hospital. These visits served as a reminder of all the good work the team had done. Away from the rushed hospital environment, I had more time to talk with patients. They were often proud to tell me about their latest accomplishment, whether it was travel, an athletic or recreational feat, or an update about their kids and grandkids, and I shared their triumphs. I also played the role of father figure to some of the younger patients, explaining the risks because, being immunosuppressed, they were vulnerable to infection. Sometimes, this meant talking to young female patients who wanted to get pregnant, helping them to weigh the risks after a transplant. Others I discouraged from engaging in activities that could undermine their newly won health, like heavy drinking or getting tattoos or multiple piercings. Some ignored my advice, perhaps out of the arrogance of youth. A few even got a tattoo on their back of a pair of lungs, with their transplant date emblazoned below. I didn't dare say it, but I thought those were pretty cool—an age-appropriate homage to lung transplantation.

I treated these younger patients like they were my own kids, and in some cases, it felt like they were. Their parents thanked me for helping to keep their kids out of the tattoo parlors or, sometimes, the bars. I cared about them deeply, and I wanted them to live long and well with their new lungs.

In our postoperative lung clinic, my team usually saw fifteen to twenty patients in the morning, and most were relatively healthy, but some were very sick. I enjoyed going to clinic and even thought that as I got older, I might eventually give up the hospital work and just see outpatients in clinic. Most days it gave me a lift to see all the patients gathered in the waiting room, many calling out to me— and sometimes even clapping—as I walked by. Each time I responded the same way: I'd wave off the applause, then take a bow, then wave it off again. The familiar routine of me being a ham was one the patients and I both enjoyed.

Tina Dahlgren was my first patient in clinic one day in 2011, a routine follow-up appointment. At twenty-five with cystic fibrosis, she had received a transplant in 2007 and had done well postoperatively, except for some hallucinations related to her medications. Later, she and I joked a lot about that, and everything else. I often told her I liked her better when she was hallucinating.

From hiking in Yosemite National Park to earning a medal in track and field at the World Transplant Games, Tina was extracting every last drop of life from her transplant. She was a bundle of energy, a free spirit, and a mentor to other transplant patients, showing them the ropes and giving them advice on how to live their lives after transplant. She often asked me if she was my favorite patient. I told her I couldn't have favorites, that all the patients were my favorite. She didn't buy it, though. The truth is I loved this girl. She reminded me of my younger daughter, Ava—no boundaries, no filters, always searching for mischief.

That day I walked into the room, throwing open the door to make her laugh. As usual, she was seated in front of the computer intended for the doctor or nurse. The computer keyboard was on her lap and her feet were up on the desk—the standard Tina position. She was trying to look up her own lab results, violating various rules about patient confidentiality. She liked to interpret her own X-rays and lung-function tests, a habit that had prompted me to give her the nickname "Doctor D" soon after her transplant.

"Doctor D. What's happening? And get off the computer." I nudged her legs with my foot.

Tina laughed, jumped up, and gave me a hug. "Come on, David, lighten up. Just checking out the old labs. Know what I mean?"

I couldn't help but laugh. None of my other patients called me by my first name, but for Tina it was natural. I sat down in what was usually the patient's chair and told her I didn't feel well and needed her help. She played right along.

"You need some time off with the Missus. Get falling-down drunk and screw all night long."

"I'll keep that in mind. How you doing?"

"Dandy. Well, not as well as I was doing. Can't climb up the mountains as fast but hanging in there."

"You're probably just getting old."

"I am not! Fuck, David, you can't even remember back to when you were my age." She was never afraid to unleash salty language, which only endeared her to me more.

"Probably right. I think I was in medical school when I was your age, never realizing that after all that hard work, I'd be stuck taking care of people like you."

"You're so lucky. You love taking care of me." She looked at me, her face turning serious. "David, if I get to the point where I need another transplant, can I get one?"

"Sure. Fine by me. Let's just order a couple of lungs up now."

"You're a dipshit. Just think about it."

"Don't worry," I said. "I've already thought about it. We'll take care of it." She gave me one big nod, stood up, and slapped me on the back.

"Way to be, Weill."

I laughed and shook my head. Then I gave her a hug.

"Alright, get outta here," I said. "I have real patients to see."

Fourteen

ater that fall, I was on rounds at the hospital when one of the anesthesia doctors asked me if I'd heard the rumor that Dr. Andrew Stevens was leaving to become the president of a major medical device company. I texted Andrew, who confirmed the rumor and asked me to stop by his office.

On my way to his office, I thought about what Andrew had meant to me over the past six years. Not only had he recruited me to Stanford—and been the principal reason I wanted to work there—but we had known each other for years prior, running into each other at meetings, sitting on national committees together, and catching up by phone. We were both guys *from* the South and *of* the South: fans of college football, the Gulf Coast, and warm weather. We often talked about the constant chill of Northern California, and I think we shared the opinion that this extended to some of the people at Stanford as well. Although we weren't best friends, I'd always felt he was a kindred spirit, someone who'd watch over me and would have my back when hospital politics heated up. He'd proven himself to be my guardian angel, keeping those who weren't happy with me off my back.

After I finished rounds an hour later, I went over to Andrew's office. I sat on his couch and started in, smiling. "You're leaving me alone with these people?" We both laughed.

Despite its long tradition at Stanford, lung transplant was not the cardiothoracic surgery department's top priority; heart surgery was. And to most, it seemed we had a solid program with decent outcomes: Why fix what wasn't broken? I disagreed, convinced that without innovation the lung transplant program would become outdated and never reach the highest echelon of quality. I wasn't settling for "decent." I was striving for "best." Or as my high school basketball coach, Billy Fitzgerald, used to say, "Don't be good, be great." I took that to heart.

But there was no point in getting into any of the program's challenges now. Andrew was leaving and any issues within the program were no longer his problem—they were mine. "Congratulations on your new position, Andrew. Thank you for recruiting me to come here. It's been quite an experience."

But not a very good one of late. Over the last few months, we continued to transplant patients at a reasonable rate. Some patients did well, but some did not—not so much in terms of post-transplant survival rates, but rather in terms of debilitating complications that would keep them in the hospital too long. I started to notice these extended stays were becoming a trend—a bad one. Each time we did a transplant I found myself wondering what outcome to expect, and our inconsistent performance made me feel increasingly on edge every time donor lungs were offered to us.

Andrew said, "You've done a great job of building the program. You put us back on the map. But the surgical team is young. Be patient with them."

"I'll try," I said, knowing that patience was not my strong suit, especially when it came to the transplant business. "We'll deal with it," I said. "Good luck to you, Andrew. I'm going to miss you."

Walking back to the hospital, I felt alone. First Johan had resigned, and now Andrew. Our surgical team had been one of the main reasons I'd moved my family from Colorado, and most of the surgical veterans were now gone, either retired or off to greener pastures. I was becoming concerned about being able to fulfill the promises I made to the patients: to get them on the waiting list, transplanted safely, and then back home to their families. This was the reason they came to see us and the reason we were in business. I was consumed by thoughts about the gravity of this, nearly all of the time. And as I left Andrew's office building that day and walked among the cherry blossom trees that lined the path back to the hospital, I had never felt the weight of that responsibility more profoundly.

In late 2012 and early 2013, more patients than I'd have liked did not do well after their transplants, which I felt was a direct result of the departure of the more experienced members of the surgical team. To make matters even more challenging, one of the younger, very talented surgeons—who was being groomed to be the surgical leader—also had decided to leave Stanford.

I finally began to admit to myself that the program I was leading—that I had overhauled, and that had occupied my thoughts for nearly every waking moment since 2005—wasn't performing as well as it could. But I needed to do more than admit this to myself—I needed to act, to come up with a plan as soon as possible.

I knew that most programs go through these sorts of phases, but I also knew that less-experienced programs like ours were more likely to have some patients who suffered complications. More seasoned teams are able to self-correct after a bad outcome, while less-seasoned teams often don't even know what went wrong or how to correct their mistakes.

I began to worry that our team was one of those not able to self-correct. I contemplated bringing in consultants to evaluate the program and make recommendations. I had provided this type of evaluation for several programs across the country, and they had always been grateful for the help. This consulting work had helped me understand all that can go wrong in a transplant program, and the steps necessary to move forward from a bad outcome. I began to draft a list of experienced lung transplant physicians and surgeons who might be able to provide this sort of evaluation for us.

Fifteen

One of the patients we transplanted during this period was Katie, a young woman with cystic fibrosis who had moved from Reno to be listed for transplant at Stanford. She was bright, determined, compliant, and desperate for the transplant. Like many with cystic fibrosis, she had been managing the disease since childhood. Her all-day regimens included inhaled medications, IV antibiotics, and respiratory therapies, with frequent clinic visits and hospitalizations sprinkled in. All in an effort to expel the putrid, infected mucous that was literally drowning her and other CF patients every hour of the day.

In our first meeting I had asked her—as I did all my new patients—what she most wanted to do when she could breathe normally. She replied she had a simple aspiration: to be a better wife to her husband, Rich. She wanted to be free from the daily grind of taking care of herself, so she could fully engage with her husband and make him happy.

Make *him* happy. I thought about her response for the rest of the day. Make *him* happy. Katie's wish was yet another example of the courage and selflessness that many of my transplant patients possessed. It made me reflect on how many of us, without a life-threatening disease to fight every day, take our spouses for granted.

I thought about my own marriage. I was a good enough husband to Jackie in the conventional sense, but there were times when I was so emotionally spent from my job that I was detached at home. With our girls I was more present, because I knew they needed me. Jackie was self-sufficient, no doubt about it, but I should have given her more of myself in those years. Time with my wife was one of the casualties of my job at Stanford, but people like Katie reminded me to do better, to be better.

A beautiful aspect of my job was hearing patients' responses to my question about what they'd like to do once they could breathe again. Their answers reminded me of what was important. It seemed these patients had the clarity of mind that can only come from facing one's own mortality.

Most didn't have grandiose plans. They didn't want to be secretary of state or run an international business. Mostly they just wanted to be normal, to be able to do the simple things without having to struggle, to embrace fully the little joys every day that most of us overlook. After their transplants, most of them would enjoy these simple pleasures much more than those of us not facing major health problems.

When a donor became available for Katie a few months later, the surgical team and I had a series of tense conversations about the quality of the donor's lungs. I thought they would be fine, and after some debate, we decided to use them. A team was dispatched to procure the organs and bring them back to Stanford.

At the donor hospital, however, the situation had changed—as it often does. The assessment of donor lungs is a minute-by-minute evaluation, and at times lungs deemed usable at one point along the way are no longer usable if conditions change. The analysis is fluid, and the best way to evaluate donor organs is to constantly evaluate new information as it becomes available.

While our procurement team was hundreds of miles from Stanford at the donor hospital, they called to express concern about the quality of the donor lungs. They were worried the lungs might have become flooded with fluid, which can happen through a complex physiologic reflex in a brain-dead organ donor.

"What do you think?" I asked the procuring surgeon. "You're there looking at the lungs." One challenging aspect of a donor evaluation is that I was usually not the one at the donor hospital examining the lungs.

"I guess they'll be okay," he said. "Should be fine, I think." He sounded uncertain, but one often can't be sure a set of donor lungs will work. An agonizing aspect of the lung transplant field.

"Okay. Let's go with it," I said. I needed to be decisive, even when I didn't feel that way.

Here was a clear example of our team's tenuous relationship with risk: The easy route would have been to turn down the lungs and abort the procedure. No one would question our judgment, and Katie would continue to wait for another donor. But she could die before getting another lung offer, and we could not ensure that she wouldn't. That's why the whole team—and not just me—spent a lot of our time walking a tightrope—if we leaned too far one way and transplanted with less-than-ideal lungs, the patient could die. Too far to the other way, waiting for the perfect organs, and the patient could die on the waiting list. As the one primarily responsible for making these decisions, this was the perilous path I had to walk every day. And night.

Too often I found myself, for the sake of a waiting patient, talking the surgeons into doing the transplant. We would have the same discussions, the same disagreements about whether to accept the donor lungs—I in favor, the surgeons opposed. It was frustrating—for them as well as for me, no doubt.

By the time the surgical team tried to transplant the lungs into Katie, they would not fit inside her chest. But once a patient's lungs come out, there's no going back. The surgical team had to figure out how to make it work with the donor lungs. They had been damaged during the procurement process, and the extent of edema (swelling) was so severe, that once the surgical team sewed them in, they could not close Katie's chest. It was like trying to close an overfilled suitcase. They had to send her back to the ICU with an open chest—never a good sign in lung transplantation.

In the ICU after surgery, while the team tried to stabilize Katie, I spoke with the lead surgeon. He looked like he had gone twelve rounds with Mike Tyson. He was sitting quietly, slumped in a chair near Katie's bed, doing his best to ignore the ICU team urgently circling her bed. The room was loud, like a subway station during rush hour, multiple conversations adding to the noise of the wailing monitor alarms. I'd already heard from the anesthesia team about what had happened in the OR, so there was no need to pry the details out of the surgeon, who was clearly exhausted.

"Tough one, huh?" was all I could say. It tormented me that after all of our efforts, Katie would actually be worse off. The surgeon took a few bites of a granola bar and didn't look up. I felt terrible for him. He'd fixed his eyes on Katie, who lay on her back, with surgical blankets covering her open chest cavity.

Finally, he said softly, "Yeah, you could say that."

"Well, let us see what we can do with her," I said. "We'll try to get those lungs to shrink down, remove some fluid with dialysis. We'll get after it."

I was trying to sound confident and upbeat, but it was all for show. He nodded glumly, seeing little reason to be optimistic.

"Why don't you get some sleep," I said. "We'll take it from here." I could tell he didn't want to leave Katie, but he couldn't provide much help at this point anyway. After a few minutes, he got up slowly.

"Thanks, David. Call me if I can help." He walked out.

After giving a few orders to the nurses and suggestions to the ICU team, I went to the waiting room to find Katie's husband. As I walked, I thought about how much bad news I'd been delivering lately. The ICU waiting room, which had once seemed like a place for smiling faces and celebratory slaps on the back after a successful transplant, had become a temple of despair, marked by tears, hushed conversations, and long hugs. I was so emotionally exhausted, both from having to be the bearer of terrible news time and time again and from a pervading sense of failure, that I hadn't succeeded at what I was hired to do: save lives. I felt that I had broken the promise I'd made to my patients to make them better.

I'd decided to become a transplant physician in spite of the fact that I knew patients would die. You'd think that, in theory, if a transplant program were struggling, the team would simply stop doing transplants or accept only "perfect" donor lungs. In practice, however, there is no way to simply press pause on a program for patients who need life-saving transplants. For our hundreds of patients, we were their only hope. They just wanted to live. They didn't care that circumstances had changed within our program—they were on our waiting list, and it was our duty to fulfill our promise to them to get them transplanted successfully.

As for the families seeing their loved ones in pain, I was left to wonder whether they should pray for another day or simply for an end to the suffering of their loved one.

The waiting room was empty except for Katie's husband, who was sitting silently, staring straight ahead. He had been there all night. Pillows and a blanket, still neatly folded, lay on the chair next to him, unused. An pizza lay in a box on the floor, uneaten but for a slice. The nurses had already told him the general situation with Katie. I was there to answer questions, give my perspective, and, hopefully, offer some comfort. I sat down next to him, put my hand on his knee, and leaned in.

"Hey, how are you holding up?" I asked.

His eyes were red but dry—like he had no more tears left. "Hanging in there," he said. "So, with Katie…what do you think?"

"She's in trouble, Mr. Carter. The lungs won't fit in her chest. They're injured, so they're really swollen and big. This happens sometimes in transplant. There are things we can do, but we'll need to work fast if we're going to save her."

And with that, the tears came. Patients' families get especially emotional when I validate their own worst fear: that their loved one might actually die. I could see him searching for something to say, but he came up with nothing. After a few deep breaths, he said, "I guess do the best you can."

"We will." I stood up and patted him on the back. "I'll come back and talk with you later."

The rest of the day I kept thinking about what he had said. "Do the best you can." So simple. So harmless. A throwaway phrase that we all use, with our kids, with everyone. "Just do the best you can." But what about when you know you're not doing the best you can, and lives are at stake? What *can* you do?

When we did our best work, made no mistakes, and a patient died anyway, we needed to accept that some things were beyond our control. The reality was that all our patients were facing imminent death. As Marty used to say, "We aren't treating the measles." Transplant may have been their ticket to a longer life, but it was not an infallible process. Regardless of whether the patients would have died without a transplant, I desperately wanted to be sure we were not making mistakes that were avoidable.

After talking with Katie's husband, I left the hospital early to watch my oldest daughter Hannah's soccer game. It was a typically beautiful day in Palo Alto, as it was for most of the year, the air crisp and not a cloud in the sky. When I got to the field, I stood with Jackie and some of the other parents, keeping one eye on the game and the other on my phone—a habit that drove Jackie crazy, understandably.

After a few minutes, I settled into the rhythm of watching the kids run around, chatting with some of the parents, pacing the sidelines nervously, and yelling words of encouragement, suddenly far removed from the hospital and its heaviness.

One of Hannah's teammates scored, and as a loud cheer erupted, I got a text from one of our nurse practitioners that Katie had died. "Fuck," I muttered to myself. Immediately my mood changed, and for me the game was over. A close friend, the father of another of Hannah's teammates, saw me looking at my phone. "Saving some lives today?"

"No. Not today."

He nodded, knowing.

"Sorry," I said. I felt badly about laying something heavy on him at the soccer field.

We both went back to watching the game.

Sixteen

Not all of our program's problems were due to issues that took place during the transplant surgeries themselves. Some patients suffered complications that were unrelated to what happened in the OR.

One day in January 2013, I saw Gilberto Vidal, a patient in the postoperative clinic who had received a transplant for pulmonary fibrosis the month prior. A distinguished-looking gentleman of Argentinian descent, Gilberto was a fascinating man, a pioneering, internationally known microbiologist. Over seventy years old, he'd nonetheless seemed to me a great candidate for a transplant because of his superb physical shape, apart from his failing lungs.

Even in the later stages of his illness, when he was tethered to his oxygen tank, Gilberto continued to dress in a jacket and tie. He would rise to greet me, shake my hand warmly, and thank me for seeing him in his thick Argentinian accent.

A month or two after being wait listed, Gilberto had received his transplant and recovered well; he was out of the hospital in just seven days. The success of his transplant made the rest of the team feel more confident about taking on older patients.

I was relieved that Gilberto had done so well for reasons beyond that he was a patient under my care. Our team needed the morale boost of a successful transplant, but what was more, Gilberto had a high profile in the scientific world. While he was recovering in the hospital, various senior members of the Stanford medical community had come to visit him, including the dean of the medical school, who later sent me a congratulatory email.

All was well until now, a couple of weeks after Gilberto had left the hospital, when he came to the clinic with his wife. He was still dressed up in a shirt and tie, head held high, but he didn't look well. I could tell he was faking good cheer.

"How do you feel?" I asked.

"Just tired, Dr. Weill," he said, with his customary formality.

Fatigue is a common complaint after a transplant. Many patients don't sleep much in the hospital or in the immediate aftermath of discharge while they are adjusting to new medications. That symptom didn't worry me.

"Being tired after a transplant is not unusual, Gilberto," I said.

He nodded slowly, seemingly trying to convince himself that my lack of concern was warranted. He looked at his wife, as did I. She stared back at him, her eyes wide open and her head tilted, as if to urge him to reveal more.

Reluctantly, he volunteered another symptom: tightness in his chest. "It's not really pain, just tightness," he shrugged.

My antennae went up. I thought of all the patients who had said the same thing just before they died—that they didn't have chest "pain" but rather "tightness" in their chest.

Any of these sensations is often a warning that a complication is brewing. Almost always, we admit the patient to the hospital to determine whether they might be having a heart attack. In screening all potential transplant candidates over forty, we do a cardiac catheterization to rule out heart disease. Gilberto's had been perfectly normal. He knew the results of that preoperative test, said now that he figured he was just sore from the surgical incision. I was inclined to agree; he did have a rather large incision. Nonetheless, I said we should admit him to the hospital to make sure everything was okay.

Most patients take my advice without much resistance, but Gilberto was a legend in his field and not accustomed to taking advice, even if it involved his own health. He politely declined my recommendation. Still, I persisted. "Gilberto, let's just admit you for a day or two. I agree it's probably nothing, but we should play it safe." I looked at his wife out of the corner of my eye; she was nodding in agreement. "What do you think?"

"No, but thank you, Doctor," he said firmly. "I'll do better at home."

I tried again. "Are you sure? Not even one night in the hospital?'"

"I'll be alright."

His smile failed to reassure me. But with that, the conversation was over. I held my hands up in surrender, gave him a smile back, and patted his shoulder. He shook my hand and walked out, slowly.

The next morning, I was sitting in my office, signing electronic patient charts, when I got an urgent page from one of my nurses. I dialed her right away, and she picked up on the first ring. "Hey, David. Did you hear?" I hated when anyone at work asked me that.

"Hear what?" I asked, standing up and bracing myself for bad news.

"Dr. Vidal is dead."

"What? Shit...Fuck!" I needed to hit something and looked around for anything that was easily replaceable. "What happened?"

She said Gilberto's wife had called paramedics in the middle of the night when he complained of chest pain and shortness of breath. He eventually suffered a cardiac arrest, and the paramedics were unable to revive him.

I couldn't speak. I felt nauseated.

After a period of silence, the nurse quietly said, "David?"

I took a deep breath in. "Yeah?"

"Need anything?"

Yeah, a stiff drink, I thought. "No but thank you. I'll talk to you later." I hung up and rubbed my face.

Fuck. I'd let a patient go home who was complaining of chest pain. I'd ignored my better judgment. I went into replay mode, thinking through all the different ways I could have handled the situation, my thoughts moving a mile a minute. *Why didn't I insist he come into the hospital? Why did I give him a say in the decision?* He was accomplished in his own field, but I was his physician. I was supposed to be treating him objectively, looking out for danger signs, and protecting him, not engaging in negotiation with him about his care. *What in God's name was I thinking? How could I have let this happen? What am I going to tell the team?*

Gilberto's autopsy a few days later confirmed that he'd died of a heart attack. In our team meeting that week, when we discussed his case, it was a public self-flogging. As I stood before the team, I felt like I was at an AA meeting. I told everyone I'd made a mistake, that I should have insisted that he come into the hospital. I acknowledged that, although he'd refused, I could have been more forceful. They didn't say a word. They knew I felt bad enough already.

It was the medical equivalent of asking forgiveness for a sin—but I was not ready to be forgiven by my team, because I could not forgive myself. We talked about how none of us had ever seen a heart attack this soon after transplant—especially in a patient with a normal pre-operative heart evaluation, which we do explicitly to prevent this sort of thing from happening. Everyone tried to make me feel better, saying that they, too, would have let Gilberto go—that he should have let me admit him.

This was unfamiliar territory. I was usually the one who played the role of priest, taking confession and granting absolution, and not the other way around. I had spent the past year concerned about the surgical team's experience level, but in this case, I had to take personal responsibility for Gilberto's death.

After the meeting, I walked straight to my office to get my bike to ride home. I was eager to get out of there. At the elevator, I was impatient for the doors to open. *Why is it taking so long?* I thought. *Hurry! One, two, three—*

When the elevator doors opened, I wheeled my bike in and jammed the button several times for good measure. Once the doors closed, I closed my eyes for a second. Then, in a sudden blaze of fury, I smashed the front wheel of my bike into the side wall of the elevator, over and over, yelling every expletive that came to mind.

When the doors opened, it occurred to me to look to see if there was a video camera in the elevator. Thankfully, there was none. I had avoided a YouTube moment.

Relieved that no one had seen me, I slinked out of the elevator, nodding at a cardiology colleague as he passed by me on my way out.

"Leaving early, Dave?" he called. "Must be nice!"

I smiled a fake smile and kept walking. "Yeah, leaving early. Life's too short." *Way too short*, I thought.

That afternoon I called my father. It was cocktail hour on the East Coast, so I found him in a good mood.

"What's up?" I asked.

"Just watching the news," he said. "Seeing what your president is up to. How's everything in the land of the liberals?" He laughed, and I smiled and shook my head. He never got enough of poking fun at California, criticizing President Obama, or me for living on the "Left Coast."

"What are you doing?" he asked. I could hear the ice clinking in his glass.

"Got out of work early. Had a rough day." I poured myself a glass of wine in the kitchen and walked outside to our back patio. I plopped on a patio chair and took a long sip, admiring the array of colors in the garden in our backyard. Jackie spent hours tending to the flowerbeds, which had grown to be so beautiful.

"Really, to tell you the truth, I've had a rough last year," I said with a sigh.

I had talked with Dad frequently over the last several months about the troubles the program was having, about patients we'd lost, and about strategies for dealing with the hospital politics. His advice was nearly always good, even if he had a tendency to suggest that I be more assertive— something he'd always encouraged. He thought most problems were best addressed by showing a stronger will. But I knew that being more aggressive at best would alienate my colleagues, and at worst lead to my unemployment.

"A patient died today," I said. "I really liked him. A famous researcher. From Argentina. He reminded me of you in a lot of ways." I stammered a bit as I walked around the yard.

I sat down again, put my feet up on a table, and closed my eyes. I tilted my head toward the sky and let the sun bake my face. For the first time in a long time, I let my facial muscles relax. But then I quickly lowered my head. I didn't want to feel good, didn't believe I deserved it. I needed to be miserable, to stand in "time out" a while longer.

"People die, David. Even your patients. Maybe especially your patients. They're pretty sick, you know," he said, laughing, reminding me of an obvious truth that I seldom acknowledged as a factor in my patients' deaths. They were *really* sick, for heaven's sake. But it was easier for me to think that I had control over the process, that all deaths in *my* program were preventable.

"Yeah, I know," I said, feeling a little better, from the wine but also because of Dad's understanding and reasonable points. I took another sip. "Seems like it's been happening too much lately. Maybe I just need a break. I should go to Florida."

"Another vacation?" This was a running joke. Every time I mentioned vacation, he would ask, as if about to go into shock, how many I planned to take.

"Yeah, another vacation," I said, playing along. "To Florida for Spring Break. Maybe I'll finally buy a house down there. So I can hang it all up, sell hot dogs on the beach, and get away from all this death and dying shit."

"You're a bit too wound up for that."

"And you're not?" I laughed.

"Well then, you're too young for that."

"Funny, I don't feel that way anymore."

"That happens, Dave. Talk to you tomorrow."

Later that night, after the kids had gone to bed, I was sitting alone in our living room looking at my waiting list. I unfolded it and read through the names: Mrs. Danbury, sixty-three, emphysema, blood type A, five foot five. *We can take a slightly larger person's lungs for her,* I thought, *maybe a guy who's five foot ten.* Ms. Coleman, twenty-five, cystic fibrosis, blood type O, five foot four. *Really sick. Saw her in clinic last week. Needs a pair of lungs—now.* I imagined a donor call for her coming to me tonight, and the process being set into motion. Next: Mr. Graham, fifty-four, pulmonary fibrosis, blood type A, five foot eleven. *He's good,* I thought. *He can wait a bit longer, just talked with him yesterday.* And then, Mr. Lundquist…

I finished going through the rest of the list and put it down on the table. And waited, willing a donor call to come for one of the patients on the list.

Seventeen

This job demands you make a hundred decisions a day. If you're good at your job, most are the right ones. Some you want to take back, like not insisting that Gilberto spend the night in the hospital. To be successful at organ transplantation, with so many moving parts, you need to avoid the unforced errors. Control what you can control.

With that in mind, I still believed it was important that the surgery department hire new surgeons. Not because those we had were bad surgeons or bad people, but because I knew we could find surgeons with more experience—an invaluable commodity in our line of work. I had spoken several times with the people in charge of hiring about our program's lack of surgical experience. Some expressed frustration at the fact that, as a non-surgeon, I was trying to make decisions about surgical matters. This was probably one of the reasons there had been no progress on hiring new surgical team members, but certainly not the only one. As usual in a large institution—in healthcare or other fields—the other reasons involved money and ego. If a new hotshot surgeon from another transplant program joined us, we would need to pay them a lot of money, which the recruited surgeon would in turn need to generate via an increased volume of patients and operations. Sometimes a surgeon is able to simply attract more patients to the hospital, but most often they take cases from the other surgeons at the hospital, which results in a zero-sum game.

And in fact, during this time period, we had interviewed experienced lung transplant surgeons who I thought would be great for the program, but the interview process stalled, never proceeding to the hiring stage.

In a conversation one afternoon with one of the senior surgeons in the surgery department, I explained why it was vital to hire a surgical leader who was experienced in lung transplantation. "We've put the current surgeons in an impossible situation, having them perform operations of a complexity that's above their level of experience," I said. "These operations are tricky, not just technically, but even more so in terms of the good judgment they require. Judgment that can only come from experience." The surgeon blankly stared at me, saying nothing.

The surgeons in any transplant program have a difficult job, dealing with many moving parts that need to go right in order to make the transplant a success: the right procurement of the donor lungs, the right preparation of the recipient, the right operation—all the while making sure the anesthesiologists are doing the right thing. My part of it wasn't easy either: picking the right recipients, listing the patients at the right time, picking the right donors, managing the patients through what could be a rough postoperative recovery, and then caring for them for the rest of their lives.

I felt confident that I understood the difficulties of a lung transplant operation as well as any non-surgeon, having made it a point throughout my career to learn what the surgical teams were up against. I'd spent time watching the surgeries and talking with our surgeons about problems they encountered in each patient we'd transplanted. In the other hospitals where I'd worked, I had worked hard to develop a mutual trust with the surgeons—something that I initially had at Stanford but was now lacking after our more experienced surgeons had left. And since trust is a two-way street, I had to accept my share of the blame for the deteriorating relationship.

Nonetheless, I wasn't going to let the program revert to how it was when I arrived, even after the departure of our three top surgeons. Too many people had worked too hard to right the ship. My team members were looking to me to remedy the situation—some of them told me so, and with others it felt like the elephant in the room. I'd had enough. I was ready to get more aggressive in seeking a solution. To sound the alarm.

I had a phone conversation with Gary Davis, a senior leader in the hospital, as I walked the building's perimeter, and asked for his help navigating the challenges our program faced.

I needed someone in the foxhole with me. But that person wasn't going to be Gary. He wanted to continue to meet, to sit around a table and discuss, to *hope* for a better outcome. His assumption was that reasonable people would, in time, reach a reasonable solution. From my perspective, we had already waited too long, and I couldn't allow it to continue.

I started to amp up, passionately providing my rationale for why we needed to act.

"Okay, calm down, David," he said. "Before you do anything drastic, let's get together with everyone—the surgeons, the administrators. Can you wait to do anything until we all meet?"

"Sure, Gary. Whatever. But I'm going to eventually do what I need to do." I took a deep breath and kept walking. By this time, I'd left the hospital grounds and reached the Stanford Oval. As I stood there, I watched the late-afternoon sun, just barely visible over the top of the mountains. The Oval was such a beautiful place, with Stanford's Memorial Church glistening at the far end and the mountains west of campus as a stunning backdrop.

As I hung up from Gary, a new call came through on my cell. It was a surgical resident, calling to tell me that a lung donor had become available for one of our listed patients.

There was nothing like a new transplant to distract me from all that was going on. But given the current circumstances, anxiety began to creep in, rather than the usual feeling of excitement I had when we were getting ready to do a transplant. But then I thought about the patients who didn't care about my uncertainty or my hesitation, who were on the list because they needed a transplant to survive. I decided to shift my focus from transplant politics to the current transplant patient, remembering to make everything about the "person in the bed."

After the surgical resident told me the specifics of the lung donor offer, I said softly, "Sounds good. Go ahead."

Back at the hospital, I went to see the patient who was about to get his transplant. Alan, the CEO of a large global technology firm, was sixty-two-years old with pulmonary fibrosis. He lived in Palo Alto with his wife, Lisa, a well-dressed woman who looked to be in her mid-fifties.

I smiled as I walked into the room. My patients and their families were usually nervous when they got to the hospital for the transplant, an encounter that had a different dynamic than when I had met them months earlier during the evaluation process. I did everything I could to put them at ease: cracked a few jokes, pumped them up with confidence, asked the patient what they would do once they could breathe well. Given our recent trouble getting people transplanted safely, this routine was hard to keep up, and that night I was worried. But it would have been unfair to convey that concern to a patient who had put his trust in us.

"Hey, it's the Renaldos!" I said in my most convincing game show announcer imitation. "Here for some trans...plan...tation!"

They smiled and laughed. He put down his iPad and she her Jane Austen novel. When he extended his right hand, I took it in both of mine.

"Hello, Doctor. How are you?"

"Really great. Psyched for you. We found you some really great lungs." I quickly scanned the reactions of both husband and wife, checking to see if my manufactured enthusiasm was contagious. It was. As though on cue, each gave a thumbs-up.

We all began to relax as I explained a few logistical details: when he would go to the operating room, how long he would be hooked up to the mechanical ventilator, how long he might be in the ICU, and when he could have visitors.

"Any more questions I can answer?"

They looked at each other. Then he asked, "Is the team ready to go?"

I nodded my head and gave them my most reassuring smile. "Oh yeah. Always ready."

The next day, I went by the ICU alone around 6:30 a.m. to see Alan before team rounds. It was just twelve hours after surgery, and he was doing well. Already out of bed and sitting up in a chair looking at his iPad.

I was happy that the surgery had been successful. Not just happy—relieved. Working in our transplant program had become an emotional roller coaster; one day it seemed like none of the patients was doing well, and the next day a transplant would go off without a hitch. The successes were gratifying but I thought too inconsistent.

As I talked with Alan, I got a text from Gary Davis: "Meeting set with all principals tomorrow afternoon. Thanks!"

I stared at the message for a few seconds while the team gathered around me for rounds. *Tomorrow will be monumental*, I thought. *How am I going to handle it? What will be my strategy? I need to think it through.*

For a moment, I pictured myself walking out onto a tree branch while a bunch of people were getting ready to saw it off. If I tried to shut us down, I would be severed from the program that I had built, that I had sweated and lost sleep over, for which I had shortchanged my family in pursuit of some elusive idea of a perfect transplant program. For a moment I was scared—of losing my job, of getting fired, of having to tell Jackie that we'd have to move again.

Well, if that's what it comes down to... And then I thought back to 1999, when I walked away from my position in Texas as an act of defiance against what I saw as medical carelessness, despite having no concrete job prospects. I was thirty-five then, newly married, had no house and no kids, just a rented apartment and a few bikes. I could afford to leave on a whim, to act on my impulses and my principles.

Now, in 2013, I was going to walk into a meeting at Stanford with similar grievances. But this time, nearly fifteen years later, it wasn't as easy to do the right thing. It meant jeopardizing my family's sense of stability. My instinct was to shutter the program and leave, and yet all I could think about were the roots we'd developed in California and the friends and patients we would have to leave behind if I chose to leave. I thought about all of our belongings being packed into a moving van simply because I felt I was no longer a good match for the transplant program I had rebuilt. The meeting with the brass here at Stanford was going to be much harder than the meeting in Texas all those years ago about the "wrong lung" mistake—partly because the circumstances were different, but mostly because I was different.

Eighteen

The meeting, held in one of the C-suite offices, would be run by one of the senior executives, a man adept at navigating hospital politics. He valued maintaining congeniality among physicians and preserving Stanford's world-class reputation. Given my tendency to express my concerns rather directly about our program, he saw me as pushy. Because he was politically powerful, I had steered clear of him, so as not to provoke him, for most of my time at Stanford.

In light of our recent outcomes, however, there was no way to avoid speaking my mind. When I did, I expected that he would respond by talking about "teamwork" and "better communication"—buzzwords hospital leaders often use when conflict arises. I had a concrete agenda, however: to convince those in charge to hire surgeons with more experience. Advocating for my patients' needs was my duty as a physician, and all I could do was hope the others in the room would hear me out.

I was mulling all of this over that day as the group started to gather in the administrative office. There were six of us, including a surprise attendee: Johan Karlsson. When I walked in, he gave me a slight smile and nodded. I hadn't seen him since he'd retired more than a year ago, and it threw me—my mind raced as I tried to understand why he'd been invited.

Then it hit me: he'd be playing the role of the unassailable respected elder, the gold standard of right and wrong.

The hospital executive in charge began by summarizing why we were there: to discuss a struggling program that was determined to right itself.

"We all want what's best for the patients," he concluded before asking each person, one at a time, for their perspective.

The first to speak, across from me, was the interim director of surgical services. In only a few sentences—he was not a man of many words—he basically said that the surgical team, although inexperienced, was good enough. Hardly reassuring, in my view, but this was basically the same stance he had taken in our previous discussions.

Putting inexperienced surgeons in situations where they can be successful means having them do only easy surgeries. But there are no easy lung transplants; even the least complicated transplant surgeries require years of skill and expertise. Stanford, as a world-renowned medical institution, could not be expected to only take "easy" patients. Nonetheless, in our team meeting we had each week to discuss potential transplant candidates, our surgical team had signed off on each of our transplant patients beforehand—not to mention that patients of similar risk were being transplanted at other programs all across the country. As in any transplant program, the risk we took was taken *as a team*, not by any one individual, including me.

The next to speak, Gary Davis, gave a bland assessment of the program, reiterating the obvious—that we were all interested in quality outcomes and that the hospital was ready to do whatever it could to help.

Then it was Johan's turn. "The surgeons are fine," he said, quietly but self-assuredly. "We may want to look at other factors." He looked right at me, unblinking.

I was stunned. Now it was clear: My colleagues were trying to blame me for our poor outcomes. I was certain that the next person to speak, one of my transplant physician colleagues, would take my side. In previous conversations, he had agreed wholeheartedly that we needed new surgeons. But in a final kick to the stomach, he said, "We have taken on more risk, and the surgeons, while not the most experienced team, are doing the best they can. We should work with them to make them better. And eventually maybe get a new surgeon. But for now, we should review all aspects of the program, including the medical side."

I laughed out loud, and the whole group looked at me. I couldn't help myself. I was smiling incredulously, doing my best to convey how absurd this had become.

"Let me get this straight," I said, seething inside, but with a smile on my face. "Our patients are not doing well because I can be a pain in the ass? Because I demand competence? Tell you what, I'll take the surgeons out to dinner and drinks, and we should be fine, right?"

I was now leaning forward in my chair, elbows on the table, looking around. "I'm trying to save people's lives here. Not sure what everyone else is doing." I leaned back. No one spoke, so I filled the silence. "And by the way, in other conversations, every one of you has said we need new surgeons. Funny how no one seems to remember that."

There was silence for several seconds. Finally, the host chimed in. "Since there seems to be a difference of opinion, I have asked Johan to conduct a thorough review of the program and to issue a report of his findings."

Johan nodded, confirming the direction they'd undoubtedly spelled out before the meeting. But I knew that having a review conducted by someone internal was a political ploy, a review for appearances only, so the group could say it was addressing the problem.

"Is that agreeable to everyone?" asked the hospital administrator. Everyone nodded except me. "David?"

"I don't think it's necessary," I said. "I know what the problem is." Then I tried to pick my words carefully. "But if we're going to get one, let's get an *external* one."

I looked back at the administration executive leading the meeting, who looked unsure what to say next. I knew it would be hard for anyone to argue against an external review—it's the gold standard, what programs do when they're struggling. After a few seconds of thought, he announced his decision. "We'll have Johan do it."

And there it was. The fix was in.

The program that I had built was falling prey to hospital politics. I was losing the fight for my point of view. It hurt my ego, but far more important, I still worried about what was best for the patients. And, I should admit, I worried about what would be next for me.

I stood up and left abruptly, speed walking furiously toward my office.

Two colleagues from the meeting called after me, but I kept walking. I heard one of them say, "I'll call him later. He's pissed."

I wouldn't advise calling, I refrained from yelling in response. *Just a suggestion.*

Back in my office, I shut the door. It was early evening now and nearly dark outside. I sat on my couch and rubbed my forehead, suddenly fatigued. On the white board hanging in my office, my daughters had scrawled messages to me during a visit to my office a few days prior. "We love you, Dad," Hannah had written. Ava's note read, "Have a nice day at work." I smiled. I was glad my two little girls didn't know what this job was really like, or what it was doing to me.

Reluctantly, I erased the messages from my daughters—in a symbolic act that eliminated any evidence of purity in the building. I closed my eyes and conjured up my father's voice. *Take control, David. You can do anything you want. Do the right thing. What do you want?*

In my lap, I held the basketball I kept near my desk, turning it over and over, feeling the familiar worn leather in my hands.

In my office, now almost twenty years later, I thought about George, the patient I'd cared for in Dallas, who struggled mightily after his transplant but was now running his family restaurant. I thought about the pride I felt, the sense of accomplishment. I missed the feelings when things were less complicated, when it was really all about the person in the hospital bed and nothing else.

Nineteen

Twenty years seemed about right. It was a good chunk of one's life. I wanted to put in my time, to have a respectable career—one long enough to do some good, but short enough for it not to destroy me. It was time to change career directions, something I'd always thought I would do after two decades, regardless of the bureaucratic fighting that had become a feature of my job more recently. No, even as a young doctor fresh out of med school, I'd already learned and seen enough to know that this phase of my career had an expiration date.

Okay, how much longer until I've been at it twenty years? I thought. I did a quick calculation on my fingers. Forty more months would make twenty years since I'd become a transplant doctor. June 2016 would be the date. *You got this,* I thought.

With a resurgence of energy after the disappointment of the C-suite meeting, I wrote on the white board in my office: 6/2016–40/20. In forty months, it would be twenty years. I sat back down on the chair and nodded, happy to take back some control over my life. But could I make it that long? It wasn't just the frustration with the hospital politics—that was separate from the main problem. I'd had enough of not being in a position to control the outcomes of the people I was treating. As irrational as it sounds to me now, I couldn't handle anyone dying on my watch.

Many times after that day, a turning point when I'd decided it would be forty more months and no more, I laughed when visitors to my office asked me what those numbers meant. I enjoyed the little secret I had with myself. In that moment, it was comforting to know that if only I could make it forty more months—ironically, about the time that I had spent in medical school—I could excuse myself from this job.

Having an exit plan opened the door for me to think about my Second Act: selling hot dogs on the beach, opening up a bike shop, maybe writing a book. I conjured up a mental image of myself as an author with an office by the sea, the sighs and whispers of the rolling ocean rather than the blaring sounds of patient alarms and bedside monitors as the soundtrack of my life.

It felt so good to think of an existence in which I wouldn't have any responsibility for someone living or dying. I may have been trapped in this skin temporarily, but it was liberating to know that I wouldn't be forever. I dreamed about what I would be like, who I could become, just like I had when I was younger and had all the choices in the world in front of me. Before it got so fucked up.

After an hour in my office, I began to feel a bit better and decided to leave for the day. Riding home, I passed Castilleja

School and Palo Alto High School. That day, as on many other days, I rode alongside kids leaving team practices and other after-school activities. Cycling down Bryant Street, a main biking thoroughfare in Palo Alto that is mostly closed to car traffic, I blended into the pack.

When I got home, my cell phone had already begun to ring before I even had my bike up the driveway. I looked at the caller ID. It was Gary from the hospital.

"Hi," I said flatly. I waited. I certainly had no intention of being engaging.

"I just wanted to talk with you about the meeting," he said. He went on to explain his position: that it was best to work together, that we should take (*I* should take) more of a team approach, blah, blah, blah. If there were a glossary of platitudes, he could have been reading straight from it. His words were hard to refute, but devoid of meaning. I held the phone away from my ear, to gain some emotional distance. He said how important he thought it was to have Johan do his review of the program. I had heard enough.

"Gary, don't you get it?" I asked. "The 'review' is for show. Johan will look at some patient charts, conclude that there is blame to spread around for things not going well, and say 'Gee, guys, just try to do a better job of getting along.' Meanwhile, nothing will change. Don't you get the position I'm in? I think we should say, 'No thanks' to the review."

"I think we need to let him do the review. Everyone wants him to do it." He was choosing what was popular over what was right.

"I think we should try to stop him from doing the review," I said. "It will only serve to validate flawed thinking. Everyone else will say, 'See? The highly reasonable Dr.

Karlsson has spoken. The surgeons are fine; the program just got a little off track. And David needs to get along a little better.' You may think it's a good idea, but I don't."

Gary said nothing but gave an exasperated sigh. "If you do anything to derail Johan's review, I won't support you," he said. "You'll be on your own."

"So what else is new?" I asked. Then I hung up.

Just then, I wondered what our patients thought of us—not in terms of our personalities or appearances, but whether they believed we would always do the right thing for them. I wondered, *Could they possibly know what decisions we were making on their behalf and how we were making those decisions?* I hoped not. Because I knew they counted on us to make their well-being our top priority, their very survival the first thing we thought of when we got up in the morning.

I wondered.

Twenty

A couple of months later, I received an email from Johan saying he had completed his review and wanted to meet with me to go over it before distributing it to everyone else. We sat down together the next day. He waited for me to speak first.

"So, you finished your report?" I finally asked.

"Yes."

This was going to be like pulling teeth. I shifted in my chair. "Great, what'd you find?"

Leafing slowly through the pages, he said, "There were a variety of problems with all aspects of the program: ICU care, donor selection, and recipient selection with older patients. There were some surgical complications, but not an inordinate amount." He leaned back, looked at me, and took his glasses off. "You can read through it. I'll give it to the others today or tomorrow."

We just looked at each other. I didn't have much to say. As I flipped through the report, I looked at the highlights: excessively long ischemia times (from when lungs are out of a donor until they are implanted in a recipient), too many postoperative blood transfusions (the result of excessive operative bleeding), some risk in donor selection, and a few higher risk recipients. In other words, all the factors that can influence outcomes—responsibility for why we were struggling shared between the medical and surgical sides.

I thanked him for the time he'd spent, and he slowly gathered his things and turned to walk out. Before leaving my office, he pointed at a picture on the wall of me riding up a mountain in France. "Maybe you should ride your bike more. Not think about this so much."

I gave him a half smile and nodded, then watched him walk out of my office. *Maybe so, Johan.* I thought. *Maybe so.*

After Johan disseminated his report, I kept my head down for a few weeks, trying to focus only on my patients. A number of people at the hospital asked what I thought of the report, but I kept my thoughts to myself. It was a détente of sorts, a cease-fire. I had already made my opinion of the review quite clear to those who needed to hear it. Plus, I was quickly losing trust in the people around me. Some saw our problems in a more balanced way—that there was mutual responsibility for why we were struggling. And whatever the issues were, I worried that any comment I made would be misconstrued, taken out of context, or sound defensive.

Staying busy with getting some successful transplants done helped ease the sting of my disagreement with the others. I realized that, given my colleagues would be at Stanford for the long haul, if I wanted to stay there to complete my twenty years in the field, I needed to learn to coexist with them peacefully.

There was a good chance I wouldn't remain at Stanford, even long enough to get to my self-imposed finish line in

June 2016. I was beginning to consider finding another job. I genuinely wasn't clear on whether I was frustrated with what was happening at Stanford or with the entire field. My skill set was in high demand, because there weren't enough transplant doctors with leadership experience to fill the positions that were open. I decided then to put some feelers out and let it be known that I was available.

Deep down, though, I was reluctant to leave the program, because in some ways I felt I *was* the program—both the best and worst parts of me. I had worked so hard to build it, and with a little help, I knew I could fix things. Even more important, I didn't want my family to have to move again. We liked Palo Alto and wanted to stay put there—maybe forever.

I thought about all the patients we had helped, the grandmother with emphysema who watched her kids play in her vegetable garden, the young kid with cystic fibrosis who learned to rock climb in Yosemite, the patient with congenital heart disease who received a combined heart-lung transplant and went skydiving three months later. We had raised the bar in lung transplant by accepting patients into our program who were out of hope, out of options, and out of time.

After mulling it over for some time, I resigned myself to staying at Stanford for a while longer, whether I was unhappy or not.

Late one Wednesday night in the spring of 2013, I sat in the ICU at Tina's (aka Doctor D's) bedside. She'd begun to deteriorate from chronic rejection of her lungs, and I had put her back on the waiting list for a second transplant.

My feet were propped up on a chair as I stared at the bedside monitor, hands clasped beneath my chin, the blips from the screen lulling me into a trance. Tina was heavily sedated, her nurse working quietly on the computer in the corner of the room. I was glad—I didn't feel like talking.

Tina had become increasingly sick in recent weeks. As we sedated her so we could put her on a mechanical ventilator, I whispered in her ear, "Not a problem, kiddo. I got this. Piece of cake. One set of new lungs coming right up." In her typically blunt way, she had told me that she was "dying like a fucking dog." And she was. She knew it and I knew it.

As I sat by her bedside, the nurses on our team would periodically come by and ask me if she was still a candidate for a transplant. All I could do was stare blankly ahead and answer yes without any further explanation. Finally, when one nurse asked me the same question again, I lashed out: "Yes! Why do you keep asking me that?" I stared her down, daring her to ask me again. I loved Tina like a daughter, and I hadn't been able to accept that my favorite patient—my kindred spirit—wasn't going to make it.

I had subconsciously decided that if I said Tina was still eligible for a transplant, then she was. And if she was, we could still save her. It was time to have a discussion with her family about the details of the end of her life, but instead I had spent my time scrambling to get her relisted for another transplant and assuring her parents that things were going to work out, that I had everything under control.

I'd known it was a long shot, and as I sat there in the ICU, watching Tina die slowly from respiratory failure, pneumonia, and kidney problems, it was clear that we would not find her donor lungs in time. Technically, she was still on the waiting list, but she was far too sick for that now.

It was time to say goodbye.

Even with heavy sedation, the effects of pneumonia were visible: poor oxygenation and difficulty removing carbon dioxide from her blood. The futility of our efforts hit me with the force of a car crash. I tried to think of another way to save her—anything else that I could try. *"C'mon, David, you fucker,"* I could hear Tina say in my head. *"Do something!"*

Doesn't it look like I'm trying? I replied to the voice in my head. *I'm not God.* I found my internal monologue was simultaneously explaining my position and begging for her forgiveness.

"Not God? That's pretty clear." I could almost hear Tina's high-pitched, nearly maniacal laugh, and imagined her red hair flying as her body convulsed hysterically.

I smiled. *Tina, you're killing me. You and all the others like you.*

"More like, you're killing us," I imagined her saying with a hysterical laugh. Tina always got the last word, even on her way to the other side.

I stood up and went to her bedside. Her eyes were closed, her chest moving up and down with the ventilator cycles. I touched her face and it felt cool—not as cold as a dead person, but not as warm as someone fully alive either. I put my hand on her forehead and then over her eyes and held it there for a moment. I leaned over and kissed her forehead. "Doctor D.," I said so softly that even the nurse couldn't hear me. Tears came to my eyes. "Sorry." I needed to leave before I lost it. It was time to go talk to her parents.

After talking with the family, there was an all-too-familiar exchange of pleasantries. "I really liked Tina," I said, and they responded, "Dr. Weill, she really appreciated all you did for her, the relationship you two had." I called Carol and told her to take Tina off the waiting list. It was the official end of Tina's rope, and I was the one who had to cut her lifeline. I felt simultaneously crushed and relieved. As devastated as I was, I was relieved to no longer be perpetuating the charade that Tina could be saved by a transplant again. It was time to face that fact that she was too far gone.

It was also time for me to face some facts about my career. Continuing to do this work the way I was doing it was not sustainable. I needed to get off the merry-go-round. I just didn't know how. I didn't think I could stop myself—transplant was my duty, my responsibility, and what I was trained and programmed to do. It was hard to imagine leaving my post, but I needed to find a graceful exit, an elegant off-ramp that would satisfy my need for a tidy conclusion. One way or another, I wanted off the roller coaster, so I could never again be crushed by a patient like Tina. That had been my life for nearly twenty years. That was enough.

I felt yanked around by the ups and downs of the job, my emotions seesawed, and all the while I had to make rational decisions for my patients. But for me, the job was no longer a pure and simple exercise in rationality. I had mastered the mechanics of being a transplant doctor—that was the easy part. But now, from an emotional standpoint, every wife was *my* wife, every child was *my* child, and every father was *my* father. And I needed to save them all.

Twenty-One

I t was a few months later, in June 2013, when my cell phone rang while I was riding my bike to work early one morning. An Atlanta area code. I answered as I kept riding.

"Hi. This is Nancy Daugherty from CNN. Is this Dr. David Weill?"

I tried to think of a reason CNN might be calling. I had been interviewed on TV a few times in the past, but never on a national broadcast, just for local human-interest stories about successful transplants we had done.

I pulled off the bike path on Palm Drive, intrigued. "Yes, David Weill here. How can I help?" I watched a few riders go by, undergraduates in Stanford sweatshirts, chatting as they sipped coffee.

"I'm the producer for Brooke Baldwin's show, and I'm wondering if you could appear on her show at noon today? It's a piece about the little girl in Pennsylvania who needs a lung transplant."

My instinct was to say yes, even though I wasn't sure who Brooke Baldwin was. I figured she must be someone who anchored during the day, when I was at work.

I knew about the girl Nancy was referencing, as I'd been following her plight on national news. She was ten years old, had cystic fibrosis, and needed a lung transplant. Unfortunately, very few child donor lungs become available in time to get kids on the list transplanted, and at the time, children did not receive adult donor lungs unless no adult could use the lungs—a highly unlikely scenario. Rather than watch their daughter die, the girl's parents were fighting for her access to compatible adult lungs, given that she was similar in size to some adults. The parents were arguing that the rule should be changed, by court order if necessary. I agreed. A donor lung is a donor lung. What difference should the donor and recipient's ages make?

"Sure. I'll come on the show." I looked at my watch, wondering how I was going to do hospital rounds and outpatient clinic before going on the air for a live segment at noon.

A few hours later, I drove to the studio on the Stanford campus where faculty did media appearances. On the way there, I called Jackie and then my father, so they could tune in. Dad didn't answer, so I waited a few minutes and called back. This time he picked up, sounding like he had just woken. I looked at my watch; it was nearly 3:00 p.m. in North Carolina, where my parents had moved some years earlier.

"Hey, Dad. How's it going?" I asked.

"Fine." He sounded horrible, his tone flat and his voice scratchy. I hoped it was because he was still groggy from a nap.

"Were you sleeping?"

"No, just lying down for a while. Umm…listening to music." I could hear something classical in the background.

"Look, I can't talk long," I said, "but I'm going to be on CNN in about fifteen minutes, if you and Mom want to watch."

After a few seconds of silence, my news finally seemed to register. "CNN? Okay. We'll turn it on."

I was no longer thinking about the interview. It was unlike my dad not to ask what the interview was about—to express no interest in something career-related. I could tell he didn't feel like talking, though, and I had to prepare.

"Okay, well…take a look. I'll try not to embarrass myself," I said.

He gave a small chuckle, but it seemed more out of obligation than amusement. "You'll do fine. Maybe call me later."

I walked into the studio, worried about my father and thinking about how I needed to get out to see him. Soon.

Once inside, I was greeted by the producer who would set up the live feed to CNN. The cameraman adjusted my tie, telling me that Condoleezza Rice had done an interview there earlier that morning. Another producer situated me at the right spot in front of the camera. Behind me, a backdrop showed the Stanford logo and a beautiful scene of the campus, the Oval, Memorial Church, and the Santa Cruz Mountains. Through an earpiece I could hear the news on CNN.

After a few minutes, Brooke Baldwin said that, next, she'd be talking with a transplant specialist at Stanford about the little girl in Pennsylvania waiting on a lung transplant. I willed myself to relax as I waited and closed my eyes, feeling the harshness of the studio lights even through my eyelids.

It occurred to me that, despite all the disappointment at work lately—and especially Tina's death—I was lucky to still be in my position. My job was weighty, had some heft to it, and now I was going to speak on national television about a story that had captured the country's attention. I reminded myself to feel grateful, to appreciate the moment, and understand that my role in this field was important, despite the current messiness at the hospital. A sense of serenity descended on me, and I closed my eyes again against the studio lights.

Those lights took me back to the fall of 1976. I was twelve, and my father was going to be on TV. My sisters and I huddled around to watch *The Today Show*, waiting for him to come on. Over the summer, the federal agency now known as the Centers for Disease Control and Prevention (CDC) had asked him to go to Philadelphia to help investigate an outbreak of a mysterious pneumonia that had killed more than twenty people in the Bellevue-Stratford Hotel during an American Legion convention.

The disease had struck rapidly and there was no treatment, since no one knew the cause. As one of the country's leading lung physicians, my father was especially well recognized for his investigations into disease causes. After a few months of work, he and others had cracked the case: they identified the microorganism causing the pneumonia, which was the first step toward a treatment for what later was termed Legionnaires' disease.

I was so proud to be my father's son that day. To a twelve-year-old, being on *The Today Show* meant you were famous. My father was nonchalant about it, but I couldn't wait to tell all my friends.

Tom Brokaw interviewed my father from New York City, asking him, "What were your first clues?" "How did the research team do its job?" "Will we be able to stop this deadly disease?" My father gave thoughtful, succinct answers. It was simple, really, he said. They'd identified the problem, investigated its possible causes, and figured out which one was responsible for the disease. He nodded slightly as he spoke, as if confirming his own words. He left no doubt that he and his team knew what they were doing. The interview ended with Mr. Brokaw thanking my father for his work on the crisis, for potentially saving many lives.

My sisters and I couldn't stop smiling. Our father was important! He'd saved lives! Tom Brokaw had just said it! I didn't want to go to school. I just wanted to see my dad and tell him that he seemed smart on TV. My mother made us go, though; she said I could tell Dad after school how well he'd done.

When Dad got home from work, my sisters dove in, sharing their impressions and teasing him for saying "Um" too many times. I told them both to shut up and told my dad he did great.

"Thanks, Davo," Dad said in our living room. He was washing down a few peanuts with some scotch. "Maybe you'll be on TV one day."

I blushed, considering the possibility. "Maybe as a pro basketball player."

"Maybe." He smiled at me and shrugged, indulging my fantasy. "Or maybe for something more important."

I nodded, wondering what that might be. It made me feel good to have a father who was making a difference, and I hoped some of his success would rub off on me.

The voice of the CNN producer pulled me out of my reverie. "Dr. Weill, are you ready? Fifteen seconds for Brooke." I opened my eyes, suddenly alert. The red light switched on. I thought of my dad, watching at home, and hoped he'd be proud of me.

The next thing I heard was Brooke Baldwin's voice saying, "I'm here with Dr. David Weill, the head of the lung transplant program at Stanford University. Dr. Weill, thanks for joining us."

I nodded and spent the next few minutes answering basic questions about the transplant process, subjects a patient's family would want to know, what I talked about every day. The interview was over in less than five minutes. It was a small event, but on a big stage. For me, though, it came down to an audience of one. As soon as it was over, all I wanted to know was what my father thought.

I called him on the drive back to the hospital.

"So? Did you see it?"

"Yeah," he said, still sounding groggy.

"Well, I hope I didn't make a fool of myself."

"No. You sounded fine."

He left it at that, and I knew I needed to do the same. He was clearly not going to give me the affirmation I sought. *But did it really matter?* I asked myself. It had gone well, and my father's opinion, or lack thereof, couldn't change that. I hung up and called my mother on her separate line. I was not seeking adulation but rather wanting to ask about Dad.

She answered right away. "Hey, baby!" she said in her Southern lilt. "You were so good!" She'd called me "Baby" nearly every day of my life and wasn't about to stop now, even as I approached fifty.

I smiled. "Thanks, Mom. It was a pretty easy interview."

"I know, but you looked so professional." She was always complimentary and supportive of my sisters and me—a welcome contrast to my father.

"Thanks, but I really called about Dad. He sounds terrible."

She sighed. "I know. He went to the doctor yesterday, and they ran some more bloodwork. They aren't sure what's going on, but we should have some results back next week." In my head I ran through the possibilities of what could be wrong. He had a lot of longstanding problems, but recently it had seemed to me in our phone calls that he was tired all the time.

"Okay," I said, "let's see what the blood tests show. Maybe I should come out there?"

"Well, that would be nice. I'm sure he'd like to see you. Seems like you're the only one he wants to talk to."

I swallowed hard and closed my eyes. "Okay, I'll set something up. Let me look at my work schedule and talk with Jackie."

"Okay, sweetheart. Talk soon."
"Bye, Mom."

When I got home later that evening, the kids were already in bed, but they had decorated the front hallway with signs and pictures. Ava had drawn a picture of a big TV with my head filling the entire space. I took a few of the pictures off the wall and flipped through them as Jackie took a seat next to me.

"The girls were so excited," she said.

"I can see that," I said. I lingered on a picture Hannah had drawn of a little girl in a hospital bed, with me at her bedside, holding a clipboard. Somehow, with that picture, titled "Daddy helping a girl get a transplant," she had managed to pinpoint so simply all that I ever wanted to do. So simple to put into words, but so hard to do.

Twenty-Two

The following week, I was in my office when the phone rang, and my father's number lit up the screen. I picked up on the first ring. He hardly ever called me; he usually waited for me to call him.

"I have multiple myeloma."

I closed my eyes. *No.*

He started to give me the details: low blood counts, an enlarged spleen, fatigue. I shook my head and tried to get myself out of son mode and into doctor mode. That would be more comfortable for this conversation.

"Dad, they need to do a bone marrow biopsy. Then chemotherapy. I wonder about a bone marrow transplant..." My mind was racing and my speech picking up speed, and many of my thoughts were nonsensical—I'd just spoken aloud to an eighty-year-old liver transplant patient about doing a bone marrow transplant despite a laundry list of medical problems.

I'm being ridiculous. I need to stop talking.

My father rescued me. "I don't know about any of that," he said. "I already got the X-rays. There are bone lesions, so they're recommending chemotherapy, but I'll have to think about it. I have trouble taking an aspirin at this point." He was sensitive to medications, despite having taken so many over the years. If a drug had a possible side effect, he'd be the one to have it. Chemotherapy would not go well, given what he had already been through.

"Okay, Dad, let's talk tomorrow. Maybe I'll come out there," I said. I felt desperate to make him feel better.

He laughed—not a full laugh, but the best he could do. "I guess I have to get cancer for you to come visit."

I relaxed a bit. He still had his sense of humor, but I could tell he felt hurt. I laughed as well, to lighten the mood. "Yeah, well, whatever it takes, right?"

Hanging up, I realized I had a lot to do. I needed to go home, talk with Jackie, and plan a trip to North Carolina. But I sat there for a long time wrestling with one fact: I was not going to be able to help my father this time. This cancer was the final straw. He was going to die soon, and no one—not even I—was going to be able to change that.

Just then, my phone rang. It was one of my nurses, Amy White. She was one of our most experienced nurse practitioners and someone I had come to trust in matters both professional and personal.

"What's up?" I welcomed the chance to talk about work, to be distracted.

"I thought you'd want to know that Sandra died today," she said.

This was not unexpected. I thought about Sandra, a young woman with cystic fibrosis who'd first been transplanted before I came to Stanford. A model patient, she had served as a mentor to other CF transplant patients. She was truly an ambassador for transplantation, and for our program specifically.

When Sandra's first transplant began to fail in 2007, we had done a second transplant. Several years later, just a few months ago, she'd developed a rapidly progressive bone cancer. Upon diagnosis, we knew—and she knew—that she would die from it. Cancer is a well-known complication of transplant; the immune suppression required after transplant prevents the body from performing its normal function of what I think of as cancer surveillance.

I hung up, thinking about what Sandra's mother, Elizabeth, must be going through. Sandra was her only daughter and best friend. After all they'd been through together—fighting the disease and facing transplant together—it seemed so unfair for it to end with her precious child losing her battle with one of the cruelest diseases, leaving Elizabeth to face the rest of life without her.

Grief, it occurred to me, was a truly universal experience. I was suddenly now not just a doctor but a son preparing for the death of one of his parents, and I was beginning my own process of grief, readying myself. And now, I felt connected to Elizabeth by a common emotion.

But no two people experience grief in the exact same way.

Over the next few weeks, my father tried without success to tolerate the chemotherapy drugs. After discussing it with my mother, he decided to discontinue chemotherapy and instead "let things run their course," as we say euphemistically in medicine. It was now August, and my sisters and I made plans to visit our parents in North Carolina.

In the years our parents had lived there, I did not visit them as regularly as I would have liked. The trip from California involved a six-hour flight to Charlotte, a short hop to Asheville, and a half-hour taxi ride to their house in a golf community in Flat Rock. After a long day of travel, I arrived in the early evening. I knocked on the back door, admiring the view as the sun set over the mountains behind their house. As I waited, I thought about how much I was looking forward to my sisters' arrival later that night. Now so spread out, our family had precious little time together. As is true with many families, it would be an illness that brought us back together.

My mother opened the door and gave me a big hug. We talked for a few minutes, and I asked her where Dad was. "He's in his room," she said. "He isn't coming out much these days. I bring his meals in there mostly."

I nodded, wondering what I would find when I went to see him. I put my suitcase in the guest room and went to the bathroom to splash some water on my face, perk up a bit. I wanted to seem alert, upbeat.

I went up to his room. He was in a recliner next to the bed, with his feet elevated. A table next to his chair was covered with electronics: a laptop, an iPad, the TV remote, a Kindle. I smiled, glad to see he wasn't too bored.

"Hey, what's happening?" I walked over to the chair and shook his hand. His handshake was weak and short. He was thinner than when I had last seen him, several months earlier, and he looked slightly yellow. I made a mental note to ask his doctor if the jaundice was from liver problems or something else.

He had the news on, like always, practically loud enough for people on the golf course to hear it. As we began to talk, he turned it down, but just a little.

"How was your trip?"

"Fine. You know. Long." I stopped, reluctant to complain. Neither of us said much. When I visited, we'd always had trouble getting into a conversational groove, even when he'd felt well.

After a few minutes, I pressed on. "So how do you feel?"

"Not very good," he said, looking away from the news for a moment. "I feel about how I look: bad." He shrugged.

I decided to bring a little levity, as I'd always done with my dad. "I don't notice any difference. I mean, you probably won't get any modeling assignments, but that's okay."

"Maybe I can be a model for a Depends commercial."

Now I smiled. "Good idea. I wonder if they're looking for someone. You should check."

He raised his eyebrows and nodded, then turned his attention back to the news.

We watched together for a while, and then he said he wanted to take a nap, so I went into the living room. My mother was at the grocery store. I didn't have much to do except wander around their big house. Adorned with pictures, books, and furniture from my childhood in New Orleans, the house looked somewhat familiar, but I didn't feel connected to it. It was like passing through a city I hadn't visited in decades. The memories were hazy, and what was new seemed to shroud the familiar.

I walked into my father's office, sat in his chair, and looked around the desk. Ever since I was a kid, his office had fascinated me: the medical journals neatly stacked on the shelves, the stereo next to rows of classical CDs, diplomas on the walls, the yellow-edged photograph of his mother, who had died of cancer when he was in college.

He never talked about her at all. I wondered what it must have felt like to lose a mother's love—something so unique and irreplaceable—at such a vulnerable time. I tried to imagine how it would have felt to lose my own mother early in my life. *It must have changed him,* I thought. Maybe that explained his aversion to intimacy. Did he think about her when he'd lie on his office couch listening to music, or sit outside at night smoking a cigar?

I left his study and went downstairs to the guest bedroom, where I stretched out on the bed and closed my eyes. I so rarely stayed still or even allowed myself time to think, but now was a good time for that. I thought about how all this would play out—Dad dying, our grief, the chaos and messiness of it all—and wondered what I could do to make it easier on my father, my mother, my sisters, and myself. If it had to happen, I wanted there to be some order to it, some elegance. I was still hoping to control some aspect of the process, so in some way things would unfold as I wanted them to. *Just think it through, David.*

One of my father's mantras was, "Every problem has a solution." That day, lying in my parents' guest bedroom, I still thought that applied to death, a process I was being forced to admit could not be controlled or managed—only endured.

Twenty-Three

I returned to California and dove into my routine: work, family, and exercise. We transplanted a few patients soon after I got back, and the patients recovered successfully. I found work made me happy, partly because it was a beautiful distraction from my father dying, and partly because I realized anew how great the job was when the patients did well.

The best distractions were the amusing interactions with some of my patients. Sam was a sixty-year-old man who, four days after his transplant, told me he was ready to go home. I thought it was a little early.

"Why the rush?" I asked.

"I want to have sex with the missus," he said with a straight face.

I laughed and glanced at my team members, many of whom were blushing. "Okay by me, but let's wait until your incision heals. Maybe a few more weeks."

"Not sure if I can wait, Doc."

The team was now giggling.

"Well, think of…think of some other way…to be together."

More giggles from the team. The patient nodded and winked, acknowledging that he caught my drift.

I left the room still laughing and shaking my head. "Who's next?" I asked one of the nurses, Amy White.

"Did you just tell that guy to get a blow job?" she asked as we walked.

"Yes," I said. "Doctor's orders."

One weekend in early November 2013, I was spending the Sunday as I normally did in autumn: watching the New Orleans Saints play football. As it became apparent they would lose to the lowly Jets, I called my dad to commiserate.

I waited for him to pick up, barely able to endure watching the postgame highlights. He answered by muttering, "They stink."

"Yep. A real clunker. But they're still going to the Super Bowl." It was something I always said—even when they had a losing record.

He laughed.

We chatted a little more, about who'd played well, who hadn't, whether the coach had called the right plays. We hung up after about fifteen minutes, and I didn't think about the conversation again. Until the next morning.

"Well, your father won't wake up."

It was a call from my mother at five o'clock that Monday morning.

I ran through the checklist in my head: *stroke, heart attack, intracranial bleed, blood clot.* The possibilities were endless, but there was no way to make a diagnosis over the phone. I told her to hang up with me and call 911.

I got in the shower, planning out my next moves.

At the hospital, Dad was diagnosed with pneumonia and sepsis, a bloodstream infection that had clouded his mental status and caused his blood pressure to drop. I was on a plane the next day.

I arrived late at night, and when I got to the hospital, I learned that hospice had been brought in. My sister Leslie and my mother were chatting quietly, and my father looked to be sleeping pleasantly. I thought back to an adage we learned in medical school: "Pneumonia is an old man's best friend." You just went to sleep and didn't wake up. A tidy exit.

I asked them a few questions. They spoke in hushed tones, though apparently he hadn't been responsive all day. We were in and out of my father's room for the next twenty-four hours, until the hospice staff told us visiting hours were over. I glanced over at Leslie and came up with the best idea I'd had all day.

"Let's get out of here and get some drinks and dinner." Both she and my mother raised an eyebrow, as if wondering whether we were allowed to leave.

While they gathered their things, I approached my father's bed and told him to hang in there. He was breathing a bit heavier than when I'd first arrived, and he looked gray. His skin felt cool. I did my usual scan, assessing him, checking his IV and the monitors.

"Dad, we're going to have a drink. I know you could use one as well, but not tonight. Not until you get better."

My mother gave me a sad smile. We all understood we were on deathwatch.

After dinner, Mom asked if we should go back to the hospital. I explained that it was important for her to go home and rest—that this could go on for days. I had seen patients hang on far longer than their families ever would have expected. Having given each other "permission" to leave Dad alone, we called it a night.

That night I slept a deep, dreamless sleep, until I heard the phone ring upstairs in my mother's room. I fumbled around, looking for my watch. *Six forty-five a.m.* I knew what this was about. *He's gone.*

Through the floorboards I could hear my mother talking, but I couldn't make out the words. After less than a minute, it was silent, and then I heard her steps coming down the stairs and into my room.

"He just died," she said.

I nodded, struggling with how to react. It struck me then how death doesn't announce itself. There's no drumroll, no lead-in music. It just happens—whether you're there at the bedside of your loved one, rushing to work on the freeway, or at home fast asleep.

We all went to my father's unit, where we huddled outside the room, as if to devise a strategy. I told them I'd go in first, then come out and get them. I didn't feel like much of an expert, though, given that this time the deceased was someone I loved. Someone I'd looked to throughout my life for answers to all questions, big or small. Someone who'd always been the barometer for how I felt about myself.

I walked in alone and went to the bedside. Dad was covered up to his neck in a white sheet. His face had a peaceful look, like he was asleep, except quieter—no deep breathing, no arm or leg twitches, no eye movement. His color didn't look much different—still a yellow tinge against a gray background. My bedside scan the night before had proved useless. There was nothing to process now, no IV meds dripping in, no heartbeats on the monitor, no alarms going off. Just silence. Nothing.

I felt empty. I longed for the release of a profound, overtly emotional reaction, to break down, kneel at his bed, and hold his hand, weeping uncontrollably. Instead, I fidgeted, wondering when I had stood there long enough and could go and get my mother and sister. *This is it,* I thought. *This is the last time I will see him.*

I'm ashamed now that I couldn't muster any other reaction. My non-reaction was telling. And concerning—a warning that I would only come to understand years later. I had shut down in response to a lifetime of tending to my patients' needs and others' expectations. I was so checked out that I couldn't even respond to my father's death "right." Despite dealing with it every day, I hadn't learned to "handle" death at all.

We spent the next few days on logistics, and I wondered how I'd never noticed that losing a loved one involves so much busywork. We shut down bank accounts, signed this form and that. And what to do with the body? Dad wanted to be cremated—he felt cemeteries were a waste of space. We tried to set that up, but could do nothing until we had the death certificate. Understandably, the crematorium would accept only bodies that had been confirmed as no longer alive. ("Think of the liability," the clerk at the desk explained, his eyes widening in horror. I nodded, thinking, *Yes, the liability—among a few other problems involved with cremating a living person.*)

I spent those few days going through my father's possessions, starting with his home office, which was his sanctuary. It revealed a lot about him—his proclivities, his habits, and his character. Legal pads lay neatly stacked on his desk, books arranged in perfect order on the shelves, computer wires organized behind the desk with twist ties, to prevent a haphazard tangle. His desk drawers were filled with office supplies, computer paper, yellow highlighters, and note pads. An unreasonable number of paper clips. I smiled as I took inventory. I guessed he'd taken some comfort in the fact that, should the world come to an end, he wouldn't be caught short on paper clips.

I next went into my parents' bedroom, feeling my father's eerie absence. On the bedside table was a picture of Dad as a little boy in Germany—before the war, before all the horror. I also found his Phi Beta Kappa keys and put them in my pocket, figuring that was about as close as I'd ever get to a college honor society.

At the bottom of his bedside drawer, I found something I hadn't seen before: a passport with a swastika on the cover. He'd rarely talked about his family. There were no dinner table stories of how the Nazis had chased them out of Germany. I had never asked about what he'd experienced, not wanting to pry. But seeing that passport made me I wish I had.

I opened it and saw it belonged to my grandmother, whom I'd never met. She was unsmiling in the photograph. *Not much to smile about, I guess.* Next to her picture was a large "J" stamped in red. And below that a list of her children: Hans Israel and Peter Israel, another official, state-sponsored denigration. Her prominent Berlin family, a line of rabbis dating back to the twelfth century, was dismissed with labels that could just as easily have said "Other." Or even, "Jew, get the hell out."

There were so many things about my father I still did not know. How did he deal with coming to a new country at such a young age? Why did he turn his back on his Jewish faith? Was it the Holocaust? *That would be enough*, I thought. Perhaps I would have understood him better if I had asked more questions.

I closed the passport and sat on his bed. My dad's life had started so differently from mine. He'd had to leave his childhood home and come to America at age five, not speaking a word of English. At that age, I'd spent most of my time eating ice cream with my friends by our swimming pool, riding bikes around town, or playing pick-up basketball. That was one big difference between us: he had been battle-tested early and survived, and for the rest of his life, he was driven to prove himself. He had been toughened by the best education: a hard life. I, meanwhile, had the privilege of not having experienced any such hardship. I was driven enough, but by a desire for his attention.

Twenty-Four

One night after I had returned to Palo Alto, when my kids were asleep and Jackie was in the other room, I looked at a Christmas picture of my family from the early '70s. My father looked young and confident in his navy blazer, crisp white dress shirt, and colorful bowtie. My mother's large brown eyes stared directly into the camera, her head tilted slightly to the right. My sisters, both in red velvet dresses, grinned mischievously. I stood next to them in a wool blazer and white turtleneck, the standard dress-up outfit of my childhood. All these years later I could still feel that scratchy turtleneck around my neck.

Seeing our happy expressions made me wonder, *Would I ever be that happy again? Are any of us ever as happy as adults as when we're children?* It's the natural order of things that our parents die, shattering our foundation, removing our sense of safety, I thought. The death of a parent launches us into the world to fend for ourselves. It signifies the true end of childhood, a ringing of the bell signaling that recess is over.

It felt like the photo was of someone else's family. I knew a page had turned.

Before Dad died, I'd long had a policy not to attend the funeral of any of my patients—as if I could suppress the feeling of failure that accompanied each death. The policy had served me well—until my absence deeply offended a patient's family member.

One beautiful morning, I was riding my bike in Portola Valley, accelerating down a long straightaway. I approached a church, both sides of the street lined with cars. Organ music rang out from the open church doors, and I slowed down to listen.

Then I remembered: today was Sandra's funeral, and it was happening in the church that I had just cycled past. Having survived two lung transplants, she had died of bone cancer while I was in North Carolina after Dad's cancer diagnosis. Her mother, Elizabeth, had invited our entire team to the funeral. As a matter of course, I'd decided not to attend.

But now, as I cycled past only by a bizarre coincidence, I felt guilty about not being there—and even more guilty for being on my bike, which might seem frivolous to those who had gone to the trouble to attend. "Sandra's transplant doctor was riding his bike instead of paying his respects," I could imagine someone whispering in the pews. I pedaled back up to full speed and rode away, glancing over my shoulder as the church receded from view.

Despite my guilty conscience, a couple of days later I was still surprised to receive an email from Elizabeth.

"Dr. Weill, I was reluctant to write you, but felt I had to," she wrote. "I know there are a lot of demands on your time, but it would have been so *appropriate* for you to be at Sandra's service on Saturday. And you didn't even let us know if you would be able to make it or not." She went on to say that many of my other patients had shown up, and they, too, had noted my absence.

I reread the email a few times, at first thinking, *How dare she say this to me? My father is dying, in addition to any number of my patients at any one time. Doesn't she know what I'm going through—and* have *been going through for my entire fucking career?* I shook my head.

But after a few minutes, I thought, *Maybe she's right. She needs me. The other patients need me.* I wasn't much use to Sandra anymore, but I could be of use to the survivors. *I need to do better.*

I pledged that day to be more available for my patients, and not just in conventional ways as I had in the past. *Yes, they need me to treat them, to be the best technician I can be, but they deserve more from me than that. I need to be more human—a* better *human.*

Patients tend to assume we doctors have mastered the mechanics of the job—that we understand what the research tells us, what tests to order, the right medicine to give. As physicians, we get that part. But for most of us, that's the easy part.

My father's death taught me that displays of sorrow, graciousness, and caring are a part of death, of letting someone go, but they are also a part of life—at least of a fully enlightened life. They are expressions of our humanity that meaningfully connect us to one another.

Earlier in my career I didn't fully understand the nuances of my profession, in those decades of watching people die after I had spent weeks, months, and years taking care of them. I tried to move on from each death the best I could, as quickly as I could, but at the end I had never been able to process fully what had happened to the patient, their family, and to me.

But I understood it now. And I was determined to not miss an opportunity to feel these emotions for my patients ever again, even if it might make the day to day experience of doing my job that much more demanding. It was the only choice.

Twenty-Five

During those same two weeks in November, I sat in my garage office, writing my father's eulogy. During the writing process, I decided I would seek out proper, formal religious training. I was still reading the Bible every day, but I wanted the context a formal religion offered, and that sense of community, of belonging. I hoped that embracing my spiritual side would foster a closer relationship with God and a sustained connection to my father.

After ten straight morning writing sessions in my frigid garage office, I was satisfied with the eulogy. Now I just had to deliver it. Public speaking was a big part of my professional life—so much so that my father used to say I ran my mouth for a living. This wasn't a typical speaking engagement, but it didn't exactly feel daunting either.

Even so, during the many hours I'd spent sitting alone in my garage office, something changed in me. With my writing, I'd said goodbye to one person but conceived another—a new, retooled version of myself.

We scheduled my father's service for the Monday before Thanksgiving. My sisters and mother did most of the organizing while I returned to the hospital and prepared for a three-month sabbatical that had been planned months before. Starting at the end of the year, I would use the time to oversee twelve international physicians and surgeons in writing the official guidelines for selecting lung transplant recipients for the International Society for Heart and Lung Transplantation. In essence, we'd spend those months establishing the criteria for what made for a good transplant candidate.

The irony was not lost on me that I'd be leading a group of international experts in these decisions after my very own colleagues had questioned my judgment. Nonetheless, the guidelines were critical and would become the gold standard for transplant programs. The project demanded time away, and after the turmoil at work and my father's death, I looked forward to a change in my routine, having the quiet time to write. But in the interim, I needed to be in the hospital, to care for patients and prepare for my absence.

Some patients had heard about my father's death, and in a role reversal I found both startling and touching, many showed their support and would ask how I was doing. Members of our team were also gracious about my father's death. Their words—especially condolence emails from those with whom I'd had conflicts over the previous year— were a comfort to me. I hoped that, had the situation been reversed, I would have had the integrity to be as kind. It was a good lesson. It reminded me to look for opportunities to move forward, to do and say the right thing, regardless of what may have transpired in the past.

A few weeks after my father's death, I flew with my family to New Orleans for Dad's memorial service. The next morning, I lie awake in the hotel room as the sun began to shine through the closed curtains of the hotel room. It seemed that only minutes had passed since the night before. Despite the lack of sleep, I was relieved the day was finally here; I knew the anticipation was worse than the reality would be.

My family stood at the entrance to the golf club to form a receiving line for the guests who had gathered. I chatted with childhood friends, their parents, and my father's colleagues, now mostly retired, who had come to pay their respects. I hadn't seen many of them in years. I was struck by how many had flown in from all over the country.

When it was time for the eulogy, I walked up to the podium. I smiled, taking a few moments to register all the familiar faces. Finally, I glanced at my wife and my kids. All were looking back at me. And then I started:

Words are difficult to find in situations like this. My father taught me many things, but not how to eulogize him....

It's easy when eulogizing someone to tick off their professional achievements, and my father had many.

As I went on, the words started to come more naturally. I strived to strike a balance between acknowledging he was a complex man and celebrating a life well-lived.

And then I braced myself for the hard part. I just needed to get through it without choking up.

I'm no expert on losing a parent, having only been at it for a few weeks. But I think it makes you finally grow up. There's a loneliness, a vulnerability that softens the heart, reminding us again that our time here on Earth is finite and that our relationships are what matter—what sustain us, and also what can sadden us. There is profound joy, though, in having people around us that mean something to us. Let's rejoice today in that. This experience had made me wonder what we would all do if today were our last day. Let's recommit to live our lives every day like it were our last day.

One final recollection: The night he was transplanted in Birmingham, he and I were sitting in his room. As he faced this big operation—the walk into the unknown—he turned to me and asked calmly, "Is there anything left you need to know from me?" I shrugged and said, "No, I don't think so." It was the best I could come up with. We resumed chatting nonchalantly, about nothing in particular, until it was time for his operation. As long as I live, I'll never forget the feeling of watching him go down the hallway on the stretcher, wondering if I would ever see him again. Well, Dad, I finally thought of a better answer: There's a lot left that I need to know from you. And we'll continue to have those conversations, privately, either in this world or the next.

I could barely get the words out. Tears dropped onto the pages I held in front of me. I wiped my eyes with both hands and tried to continue, starting and stopping, then starting again, after a deep breath.

Dad, and finally, to you:

Since you passed, just nineteen days ago, I've had an image in my mind of where you are now: with your feet up, holding a scotch, with the classical music cranked up, watching the Saints head toward another Super Bowl. Where you are, the suffering has ended, the days are brighter, tranquility has come. A beautiful picture indeed.

See you one day.

Once the ceremony was over and the last condolences were accepted, my extended family wanted to go out to dinner. I just couldn't do it. I was thoroughly spent, emotionally and physically. I asked Jackie if she minded staying in and eating dinner in the hotel, just the kids and us. She agreed. We had a relaxing night in the hotel room, eating room service and watching cartoons in our pajamas with the kids. It was perfect.

When I returned from New Orleans, I started my sabbatical, diving into the work on the transplant guidelines. I needed to go through twelve hundred medical articles and summarize the more important studies—an ambitious task in only three months. I welcomed the distraction, though, and it crowded out some of the sadness over my father's death.

For the first couple of weeks, I sequestered myself in my garage office, reading and writing for hours at a time. Around midday, I would leave my bunker and take a walk with Jackie and our dog, happy to talk about anything other than my grief. I wanted to process it but was still developing the language, the emotion, the vulnerability. Jackie didn't force the words out of me but instead waited patiently until I was ready.

After a few weeks of this, I slowly but surely began to lose my mind. I'd wander around my garage, looking at a picture or tossing myself a baseball. I felt alone. I'd turn on the TV and watch the stock market ticker scroll by on CNBC for a few minutes before turning it off. I felt guilty wasting time when I should be working. I missed the hospital—well, at least the structure and the human contact—the patients who needed me, the team that relied on me. I hated to think about the program going on without me, just a few miles away, while I was stuck in my dark office, reading article after article.

Soon, I started going into my office at Stanford to write instead. When colleagues asked why I was there, I made up excuses, saying I was meeting with the medical school librarian about "research." I couldn't tell them why I was really there: because I couldn't stand to be alone.

The time of contemplation imposed by my sabbatical served to reveal that my world had become too complex, too difficult. I found I could no longer tolerate this void. It felt like a hole in my soul. I was desperate to simplify, to get back to the basics of what we're all meant to do in this life and why. I needed a sense of purpose and clarity that I'd never had growing up.

Throughout my marriage to Jackie, I'd witnessed her devotion to the Catholic Church and the calming effect Mass had on her, with its flowing rituals, the standing and sitting of the parishioners, and the rhythmic prayer recitals, commitments made in unison for all to hear. I'd been thinking about religion for a long time, and specifically how it was missing from my life. I liked the idea of religion as a way to get closer to my wife and my two baptized children. So rather than adopting the Judaism of my father's parents—a religion he himself had never embraced—I made plans to convert to Catholicism.

One morning I sat at my desk, staring out the window. I had an awareness that I was changing—that this kind of work was not the same for me anymore, and perhaps it never would be. *If I'm going to continue to do it,* I thought, *I need to figure out a way to deal with this deep sense of loss. Otherwise, it will continue to crush me—more than it already has.*

I turned to my computer and Googled "Rite of Christian Initiation of Adults."

Soon my sabbatical was over—the writing project successfully completed—and I went back to work full time. On Monday evenings, I would attend RCIA classes at St. Albert the Great Catholic Church near our home in Palo Alto. I had to hustle out of the hospital, stopping briefly at home to eat something and check in with my family before running out of the house with my course syllabus to get to class in time. I would read the material over the weekend, carefully highlighting the most interesting passages—with a yellow marker like the ones my father used.

The RCIA program directors, a married couple named Seth and Mary, co-led the group with our pastor and our deacon. At the first class they introduced themselves one by one to the church newcomers and their sponsors. I learned that those going through the Catholic initiation process were required to have a sponsor, someone to offer advice and guidance about the customs and rituals of the church. Jackie would be my sponsor, but she couldn't make the Monday meetings, since we didn't have anyone to watch the kids. Each week, I would bring home my questions about the faith for her and I to discuss.

Mary had explained that each session would cover a different topic, such as who is God, what Catholics believe, the Ten Commandments. I had shied away from these sub-jects in the past, having lacked any religious framework with which to grapple with them. But I was excited to engage them now.

As we sat around the table that first week, they asked each of us to explain why we wanted to become a Catholic. While I was waiting for my turn, I thought back to my childhood, to the moment that determined my life's secular course.

One lazy Saturday afternoon when I was nine, I was lying in bed with my basketball, practicing my shot. My 8-track cas-sette player was playing the new Paul McCartney and the Wings album, *Band on the Run*—the volume turned down low so I would be able to hear when my parents called me. They had asked my sisters and me to meet with them indi-vidually in the dining room in order of age, oldest to young-est. I was last, and had been waiting for what felt like a long time already. *What do they want to talk to us about?*

My sister Leslie, who was twelve at the time, came to stand in my doorway. "Your turn," she said.

"Was it bad?" I asked. "Are we in trouble?" She shook her head no and gave me a punch in the arm before I ran upstairs, taking two steps at a time.

Our dining room was upstairs, as was our kitchen—a common setup in old Louisiana homes because of the possibility of floodwaters coming over the levees. When I reached the top of the stairs, I put my basketball down on the landing—my parents hated it when I brought the ball into the dining room—and went in.

The room was formal, with creaking hardwood floors, antique furniture, and a long table in the center surrounded by eight upholstered chairs. Underneath the table was an oriental rug that was more than a hundred years old. Overhead hung a chandelier from my grandfather's antique collection, with a few cobwebs stretching between the candleholders. My father sat at the head of the table, my mother next to him on the side. When I came in, he gestured to a chair opposite my mother. I sat down.

"Your mother and I have been talking," he began, "and we want to know whether you want to go to synagogue regularly." For some reason, in a family that wasn't particularly committed to any religion, the default house of worship had been a synagogue on the rare occasions when my parents felt it absolutely necessary to inject some religion into our lives. Mostly, our house of worship had been the Superdome where the Saints played on Sundays—something that we were all committed to, except my mother who preferred her own quiet time while the rest of the family obsessed over the fate of the dreadful Saints.

He continued. "Is it important to you? Or are you just going to complain about it each Saturday?"

I did complain about it whenever we went—but what kid didn't complain about going to church or synagogue? My feet dangled above the floor—our dining room chairs were far too big for a child—and pondered my dad's questions. I was astonished that my parents were asking my opinion. My nine-year-old brain began to process: *Is this happening? Are my parents really making this religion thing my call?*

My father stared at me, waiting for an answer. I thought about it for a second. Let's see: *Waste precious weekend hours in a neck-scratching turtleneck and blazer, or be allowed to play basketball, watch football, and hang out with my friends all day? Was this even a serious question?*

"No," I said slowly, trying to pretend that I was giving the question some serious thought. "I guess I'd rather not go. I think I'm okay without it." I sat there, expressionless, and waited.

My parents looked at each other.

"Okay, that's it," my father finally said. "You can go." I learned later that my sisters had given the same answer, an instance of rare consensus for us.

I leapt out of my chair before they could change their minds. I picked up my ball at the top of the stairs before running downstairs and out the door to my friend's basketball court around the corner.

To this day, I don't know why my parents let us kids decide whether we would practice religion as a family. It was especially out of character for my father, who didn't even solicit our opinions on trivial matters like where to eat dinner. I wondered in retrospect if his own childhood experience with religious persecution—being run out of Germany as a small boy, watching his father being hauled off to a concentration camp—contributed to him supporting us in making our own religious choices.

Or maybe the idea to consult us came from my mother. Raised as a Southern Baptist in Selma, Alabama, she went to church, as she put it, "any time the doors were open." A way of life in much of the South, her faith was perhaps not as well suited to life in a predominantly Catholic city like New Orleans.

Regardless, they received unanimous agreement from the three of us—who tended not to agree on much. But I had come to regret the absence of formal religion in my adult life. Agnosticism became uncomfortable for me as I grew older, especially when I saw so many, including my wife, derive meaning from their faith. I longed for the sense of community religion provides, for the belief in something bigger, a way to make sense of tragedy. I sought a closer bond with both my family and with God. I was no longer satisfied spending Sunday mornings riding my bike while my wife and kids went to church without me. It didn't feel right anymore.

Twenty-Six

O ne day in January, I was working in my office at Stanford when one of the young doctors on the team, Tyler Flynn, asked if he could talk to me about a patient. A former trainee, Tyler was my closest friend on our team.

Patrick was thirty-two, a cystic fibrosis patient on our waiting list. He had a pregnant wife, which made him a bit unusual in that that many CF patients—men in particular—are sterile. He was easygoing, eager for a chance at a transplant. When I asked why he wanted one, he said simply, "Because my little girl needs a father." As his time on the waiting list had dragged on, he'd become progressively sicker and been frequently admitted to the hospital with pneumonia.

"Hey, boss," Tyler said, standing in the doorway of my office. As he geared up to discuss the case, he fiddled with his lab coat, his eyes darting around the office.

"I think Patrick has gotten too sick to transplant," he said. "The risk would be too high, even if we found lungs for him today."

I shook my head, knowing what was next for me: another tough conversation with a family that had run out of time. "Did you talk to the family about taking Patrick off the list?"

And letting him die? It was the reality we both knew but did not say aloud.

"Sort of hinted at it," he said. "The family really wants to hear it from you. From someone wise. And old." We both laughed a little, but not lightheartedly.

"Yeah, and getting older by the minute." I sighed. It was my responsibility; patients' families did want to hear the news from me. It was also the natural order of things in our business; when I was younger, the older guys had delivered most of the bad news. "Okay, give me a second. I'll meet you in the ICU conference room."

While Tyler went to get the family, I sat for a minute, thinking about my own loss and the grief I was still feeling. I didn't know what to do with it or understand how I was supposed to feel or act. Being in the hospital was the best tonic I'd found since my father's death. But up to now I had avoided any difficult interactions with patients' families. I didn't know what to expect about this discussion with Patrick's family. *Will it feel different? How will it affect me?* I decided to just get back on the horse, ignoring the scrapes and bruises. I pulled on my white coat and went down to the floor with the ICU.

The family was gathered in the family room adjacent to the ICU. I'd had hundreds of conversations with families there, none of them good. It was barely big enough for more than two people, with the typical dim lighting and drab furniture, and boxes of tissues scattered throughout. When I met with large families in there, we crammed in extra chairs from the ICU waiting room so tightly we couldn't close the door.

I sat down with Patrick's wife, mother, and daughter, Anna, who looked to be about four years old. A soft smile on my face, I pulled my chair closer to his wife, who was quietly crying already.

"Patrick has gotten much sicker, as you know," I started. "Our team is wondering if he is still a suitable candidate for transplant. At times, patients on our waiting list get so sick that we can't do a transplant because it would just be too risky." I paused. "I think Patrick is now at the point where we can't transplant him safely." I stopped to let the news sink in.

His wife began to cry more loudly, clutching a tissue in both hands and wiping tears away. I looked at Patrick's daughter, who was busy drawing a picture in a notebook, oblivious to the meaning of a conversation that would forever affect her life.

"So does this mean you're taking him off the list, that he can't get a transplant?" his mother asked.

I looked at her. *Fuck, I hate this. I'm in this profession to save people—to win—not to give up and say, "Sorry we can't help you this time. Have a nice day."*

I turned away from Patrick's wife and took his mother's hand in mine. "No, we won't be able to transplant him," I said. "I'm sorry, but he's just too sick."

She withdrew her hand and reached for a tissue. Then she just looked at me, silently wiping away the tears. I felt tears running down my own face. *I'm their doctor, and I'm crying right here with them, feeling their loss.* I realized that from now on, losing patients would be even harder, would hurt me more deeply.

No one said anything for a few minutes. Finally, I looked down at Anna, who had finished drawing her picture. She got up to show it to me, standing with her little hand on my knee. I remembered my girls at her age, how they were so proud of every picture they drew and needed to show me right away. I looked at her and smiled.

"Hey, show me what you did!" I said trying to stop the tears.

She handed me the notebook. It was a picture of her, a stick figure, with her parents holding each of her hands. Above it, a cartoon sun shined rays of light all the way to the ground.

I felt more tears coming but did everything I could to choke them off. "That is so good, precious," I said. "You're such a good artist." I squeezed her shoulder gently, near her neck, as I did with my girls all the time. She laughed and squirmed, ticklish.

I stood up and gave the mother and wife quick a hug. As I was leaving, I looked back at Anna, who had already started drawing another picture. I hoped she didn't understand what was happening, that she could keep drawing pictures of the sun until she was old enough to understand that people—including her father—die for no good reason. It's just part of life. If she could somehow accept that, she'd be better off than most. Better off than I was.

Patrick died two days later. The day after that, my rounds with the team brought me to the ICU. Our first patient was Fred, a sixty-three-year-old wealth manager who suffered from emphysema. When we'd met for the first time three or four months earlier to talk about the possibility of transplant, I'd asked him my usual questions about his family, his interests, and his work. Throughout his career, he said, he'd sat at his desk day after day, chain-smoking as he watched the stock ticker crawl across his computer screen. When I told him the emphysema would kill him if he didn't get a transplant, he took the news in stride. "The cost of doing business," he said.

I found myself thinking about the cost to me of my business of lung transplantation. Mine took a less perceptible toll than emphysema, with its telltale smoker's cough. Mine was an overriding sense of guilt about the patients who had died—the sense that I'd reneged on my overconfident promises to patients and their families to save lives.

I was aware when I walked into Fred's room in the ICU that it was the same one where we had all had to say goodbye to Patrick just a few days earlier. He was sitting up, watching CNBC, looking strong just twelve hours after surgery. I could not shake the haunted feeling I had as I greeted him. *Even just a few years ago I would not have let these thoughts linger*, I thought. As much as I tried to focus on the very-much-alive patient in front of me, who was doing well after his transplant, I couldn't stop thinking about the one I'd neglected to save.

I tried to regain my focus and maintain my composure. "Hey, Fred, what's the word, my friend?"

He muted the TV. "Doing great. Piece of cake," he said.

I smiled and looked at the team standing behind me. "Glad it's going well. It doesn't always." As we shook hands, I knew what was coming next.

"When can I get out of here?"

"We'll send you out of the ICU today," I said, turning to walk away.

"No, I mean, when can I go home?"

"Soon enough," I said, turning back to him. "In the meantime, enjoy the food." He laughed.

"Okay, but let's move it along!"

Normally I would have stuck around and chatted with a patient who'd done so well after a transplant, to share in their joy and relief. But now that my father was gone, the cumulative deaths of so many others had finally caught up with me, and I couldn't enjoy it, even when things went well. Grieving for my father had opened floodgates of grief for hundreds of patients I'd lost throughout my career. Now that grief had "caught" me, I felt it attacking me from all sides.

The grief was beginning to eat away at the sense of fulfillment my work had always given me, robbing me of any of the good emotions that had attracted me to the field. I was forgetting about the transplants with positive outcomes, brushing them off, depriving myself of happiness or pride. Instead, I was focusing only on the bad outcomes, the failures. This was creating an imbalance that served as a form of self-destruction. It was not all that different from smoking cigarettes, only without the pleasure of sitting with a morning cup of coffee, inhaling deeply, blowing out rings of smoke, and watching them rise slowly toward the clouds.

I envisioned the emotional reserve of a doctor to be a sheet of paper: When I began my career, it was large and intact. The first patient death tore a little piece off one end, and the next one tore another, followed by another and another. Once the hundredth death rolls around—by which time I was a father, and about to lose my own father—it tears off a disproportionately large piece. I could feel that last piece float to the ground, and I knew it was gone for good.

Once it's gone, so is your emotional and mental capacity to lose another single person—to watch it all over again, to sit in that waiting room with one more family. You just can't do it anymore.

The popular term for this is physician burnout. Recent research links burnout to alcohol abuse, depression, suicide, and poor interpersonal relationships. The syndrome—whatever you call it—affects *half* the physicians in the United States. For the myriad physicians who experience this, there are likely whispers in the hallway among their colleagues that Dr. Whoever has "burned out." But the label should be different. I'd label it "physician humanity." I'd say to the doctor, who I'd imagine might feel ashamed or even paranoid, as I did at times, "Congratulations, they just called you a human being. How do you plead?" Because these emotions are unavoidable, and I'm not certain they should be avoided if we're to do our jobs well—it's part of being in a caring profession, one that would benefit from giving its practitioners the freedom to speak openly about how they feel about the losses, about the pain. *Our* losses, *our* pain.

I was trained as a doctor to avoid these types of emotions altogether, and as a result, I was now paying a price. The fact is that the entire field is paying a price and finally recognizing and addressing the problem—even if only acknowledging it as something we need to deal with rather than deny it is happening. We have started to tell our young doctors—I certainly tell them in my current capacity as a consultant for transplant programs—"Feel what you feel. Share it, acknowledge it as valid. Come out of the darkness with your pain."

That is the start of *healing* our physicians—for their sakes, their families', and their patients'.

As I started to make my own emotional and mental health a bigger priority, I began building my Monday routine around my RCIA classes. I would rush out of the hospital to get to the church by 7:00 p.m. And for the next ninety minutes, I would do something exceptional (for me): keep my phone off and take a break from the madness of my work life.

I came to grow fond of the people in the group. We came from various backgrounds and had different reasons for wanting to become a Catholic. One young couple from South America wanted to get married in the church "in front of God." Another young mother had married a Catholic, and when their family had fallen on hard times, she had turned to her husband's church for comfort. A man working in the technology industry, a recent immigrant from China, had an evangelical background.

And then there was me: I had emigrated from Louisiana, a place where there are no counties, only parishes; where my football team was called the Saints; where there were Catholic schools or churches on nearly every corner. I had lived a life that ran parallel to Catholicism my entire life, but I was oblivious to its influence that was all around me.

And yet now here I was, just a person taking comfort in religion, like so many before me had. I had found my way there not just to alleviate my own confusion and existential angst, but because I knew doing so would bring me closer to the people I cared for most—Jackie and the kids, who were already in the lifeboat, ready to throw me a life preserver.

Twenty-Seven

A few months later, my sisters and mother and I headed to our house in Florida to spread my father's ashes on the beach. Jackie and I had bought the house on the Florida Panhandle only a few months before my father died. Being too sick to travel, he never got a chance to see it, but in many ways, having a house there connected me to my childhood and my many memories of visiting the area when I was growing up. The long days at the beach, racing in and out of the warm Gulf waters, riding waves in with my father—it had been an important spot for us—and now it was for my family as well. It meant being together, it represented a lightness, an unburdening that we couldn't get anywhere else.

The evening in March when we spread my father's ashes turned out to be windy, cold, and clear. We made the short walk from our house in Rosemary Beach to Boardwalk D, where we had decided to let the ashes go. His remains, oddly, fit in a plastic bag the size of small trashcan liner. With a glass of wine in one hand, I took the bag out of the fancy box the funeral home had given my mother. My sisters and mother each had drink in their hand as well—just as Dad would've wanted it.

The bag was surprisingly heavy, the ashes dense like coarse sand. As I walked toward the boardwalk, I thought about the strangeness of carrying a parent's remains in a bag. After a lifetime, this was all that remained of my father's physical self. I tried not to linger on that thought long.

Once we reached the stairs leading down to the beach, we debated for a minute about where exactly to spread the ashes. Ultimately, we decided to spread them over the large sand dunes just below. I looked at the water, listened to the sound of the crashing waves mixing with the squawking of the seagulls gliding effortlessly above us. The sun was setting against the horizon. I took a deep breath and admired the view. It was so beautiful. I was glad we'd picked this spot. My father would have liked the location we chose for his final resting place.

I put the bag on the stairs, tore it open, and stared into the ashes. Some were gray, some black. I thought about which parts of him would be which. Then, forcing myself to stay on task, I lifted the bag and began to dump the ashes over the railing, watching some float gently to the top of the dunes while others fell more quickly, straight down into the sand below.

When I was almost done, the wind shifted suddenly and a strong gust hit me right in the face, filled with a good bit of my dad's ashes. I was covered—my sweater, my hair, the back of my throat. My sisters and mother started laughing as I turned back to them, looking like I was covered in soot from rolling around in a fireplace. I can imagine Dad was laughing, too. *Nice job with the bag, Davo.*

For the first time in months, I laughed with my whole body, wiping the ashes off my face, shaking them out of my hair. I was still laughing as we turned back toward home.

A clear morning in late fall. I was up early, swimming laps in the Rosemary Beach community pool. Later that morning, our family would fly back to California. I wasn't looking forward to going back—either to my life there or to leaving behind the uncomplicated beauty and respite of our beachside sanctuary.

I was enjoying the solitude of the early morning, the magnificent quiet of a morning swim. About halfway through my swim, I took a break, leaning against the side of the pool to catch my breath. A young father with his two boys, both seeming younger than five, had come into the pool area.

I recognized the kids' pool routine from when my daughters were that age: get out a bunch of floating toys from a large bag—more suited for a long trip abroad than for a visit to the pool—throw all the toys in the pool, strap on the goggles, and *splash!* They're in. Then they scream at the top of their lungs for their father to join them.

Sadly, I also recognized the dad's routine: sitting in a deck chair, glued to his phone, answering messages, talking, redialing. Busy, even on an early Saturday morning in a beach town. The kids yelled some more for him to join them. He didn't look up from his phone. I knew it only too well. *Can't right now; let me get some of this done.*

Agitated. Distracted. Me.

I watched all of this play out from across the pool, one minute turning into five, then ten minutes. Without saying a word—instead willing it with my mind—I begged him to put down the phone, but he didn't. The kids called out for him some more. He took another incoming call.

I started swimming again, sluggishly. I had rested too long and was now slow to get going. As I continued to swim, I continued to think about this young family. And mine.

Part of me was sad. I had been that father. But another part of me—the irrational part, the part I knew I needed to suppress—wanted to get out of the pool, go over, knock the phone out of his hand, grab him by the shoulders, and yell, "Don't you get it? Get a clue!"

But I didn't. I kept swimming, knowing that each of us has to learn the toughest lessons on our own, once we have made the space to work it out in the quiet of our own mind.

When I finished my laps, I got out of the pool, toweled off, and looked around. They were gone.

Twenty-Eight

I n April, my RCIA classmates and I were scheduled to
be baptized at the Easter Vigil. Leading up to the big
event, we were all eager with anticipation, asking detailed
questions about what the ceremony would be like, what we
should wear, whom to invite.

During the service, I waited by myself in a small room
in the church. It was musty and the walls were covered with
books, all related to Catholicism. I sat on a small bench and
looked up at the stained-glass window as the sun streamed
in, warming my face.

I closed my eyes, reflecting on how much had changed
over the last few months. My father's death had been the
catalyst for my awakening; I now viewed my job differently and saw it as a toxic addiction that had hurt me badly
without my even realizing it. I needed to get away from it,
to suppress the anguish associated with my job. I thought
about the patients we had lost—the deaths I had long felt
personally responsible for. Finally, after all these years, those
feelings of supreme responsibility were slowly eroding. I
understood that I wasn't the central actor in the transplant
universe anymore, that I couldn't control life or death. I

now believed a higher being was in ultimate control of that. I smiled and crossed myself, feeling relieved and at peace.

I wished I could have stayed in that room for hours. Then Mary, the member of the congregation who was helping with my baptism, came in and said it was time to go inside the chapel. I got up, put my hand on her shoulder, and walked inside the church.

Prior to my religious journey, I wasn't someone who believed that finding religion was the way toward a better life. But for me, something did change that day. Getting baptized and developing a relationship with God were important parts of the puzzle for me, leading me to a greater understanding of who I am—the good and the bad—and of my place in the world.

Going forward, the tapestry of my life would always include religion. It made me feel whole and connected me to my family and community. It's not that I was a terrible person before finding Catholicism. I'd just been lost.

At the end of that important day for my family, I found a letter Jackie had left in my home office.

Dear David,

There have been so many times in our marriage I have been proud to be your wife, but this is the brightest path we have ever journeyed together. We as a family have a wonderful long life ahead of us, and we look forward to your hand joining with ours in the Catholic religion. It is a journey I will cherish.

Love you, and so proud of you,
Jackie

I reread the letter and closed my eyes. I had been blessed beyond belief for so long—my wonderful wife, the support of my friends.

I had just finally begun to realize it.

My spiritual transformation led me to rethink my entire career path. Several options had been running through my mind in recent months, since I had completed my religious conversion: resigning outright and never coming back, asking for a leave, or requesting another sabbatical—my second in two years.

Unfortunately, there was no easy mechanism that would get me out of there just because the job—really the career—was getting to me. I knew it wasn't just a bit of burnout that a couple of weeks on the beach could fix. No, I was burnt beyond recognition, crispy. Emotionally spent from twenty years of watching people either live or die under my watch, seemingly at random.

Sabbaticals are a nice perk of university jobs, a consolation prize for putting up with the politics that goes on at some of these places. They are sort of like a mini walk-out, to see how it feels to wear the clothes of a different life. The last time I had taken one, over a year earlier, it had been to write the transplant recipient guidelines. Less grand this time, and harder to explain to those around me, I would take this one as an experimental hospital exit.

At some point I had done enough deliberating. It was time to make it official. I asked Gary Davis if we could meet.

I walked the two floors of stairs to his office slowly, trying to think of what, exactly, I wanted to tell him. In those five minutes, I decided to ask for another sabbatical. But I knew I needed to be prepared to answer questions about what I planned to do during my time away. This is what was still hanging me up, as his office got nearer and nearer. *Go to another institution and work with their transplant doctors? No, that defeats the purpose of getting away from it all. Plus, I can't leave Palo Alto for an extended period with a wife and two kids. Do some research at Stanford? No. Not interested. Work with a venture capital firm?* A few had contacted me to help with their medically oriented investments over the years.

No, not now. I want quiet time to sort out what I'm feeling and what I want to do with the rest of my life.

It came to me at the bottom of the stairwell near Gary's office. *I'll write a book.* I'd always wanted to do it.

It was a daunting task, but I wanted to try it. *Maybe about my experience as a transplant doctor. And about Dad, my father and my transplant patient. More.*

I kept walking. *That's what I'll go with.*

I knocked on Gary's door, and he waved me in and I sat down. He just looked at me, waiting for me to start.

"I wanted to talk with you about taking a sabbatical," I stammered, still unsure of how this was going to go. He nodded and smiled, so I continued. "To write a book. Maybe six months…." I looked past him, out the window.

He smiled and nodded again. *This is going better than I expected.*

"Sure," he finally said. "Thank God. I thought you were coming in here to tell me you were leaving for good."

I smiled. *I thought about it, my friend.* Then I started laughing, feigning that the suggestion that I would walk out on my job, on the program that I had built, was an absurd proposition. "No, not leaving forever," I said, trying to get a handle on what it felt like to laugh at the "silliness" of that. "Just want to get a book written."

I looked at him, trying to judge his reaction. He just kept looking at me. "I look forward to coming back," I said, disingenuously. *I don't exactly know what I look forward to doing—maybe coming back, maybe not.* In some ways, the relationship I had with my job felt like a bad marriage, each one looking at the other, wondering who would call the divorce lawyer first.

"What are you going to write about?" Gary asked. "Will it be a medical book?"

"No, just about my experiences as a transplant doctor. And maybe my experience with my father getting a transplant. Lots to say, I think."

"Well, good. Sounds interesting."

We got up and shook hands, and I walked out of his office.

I was getting out of there in less than a month. No Stanford, no transplant patients, no young people with cystic fibrosis on the waiting list. I felt thirty pounds lighter and nearly skipped back to my office. I was going to get my act back together, get some time away from this place. *Who knows? In six months, maybe I'll be healed, maybe I'll want to be back, full throttle, stomping around the hospital. Or maybe I won't.*

Twenty-Nine

As the summer of 2015 approached, we made plans to spend time in Rosemary Beach while I was on sabbatical. It was time to do some serious thinking about my future, and I knew I could do that in Florida. My identity was still so wrapped up in my job that it would require a lot of time away to remember who I was outside of work.

We arrived soon after school let out in June. It was an idyllic time. Most mornings, I woke up early and went out on the Gulf on my paddleboard. The beach was usually empty, except for a few early birds taking a walk. The water was clear, and the marine life put on a show—dolphins swimming around my board in small groups, red fish darting about, sea turtles gliding around. The serenity of those mornings was unparalleled.

The best parts of the summer were the times with my kids on the beach—swimming out to the sandbar with them, just like my father had done with me on the same stretch of beach forty years earlier, and diving twelve feet down into the warm green water to collect sand dollars off the Gulf floor.

It was so quiet at the bottom, just me and my girls, far away from my life in California and all its complexities. The three of us would rise up and burst above the water, out of breath but laughing hysterically, our hands filled with sand dollars. And in the distance, back on the shore, I could see the dunes near Boardwalk D, where we had scattered my father's ashes. I imagined him giving me a thumbs-up. *"Race you back to the shore, Davo. See if you can catch me."*

After our day on the beach, I looked forward to going to the local seafood market each afternoon to pick out the day's meal. They got to know me there—the same guy behind the counter would always ask, "What can I do for you?" I would always answer, "Make another day like today," before making my biggest decision of the day: fish or shrimp.

We would grill the seafood on our patio, the kids running around the backyard, me tending to the food, beer in hand. After dinner, Jackie and I would talk or watch a movie, before I drifted off into a sleep that was sounder than any I'd had in years.

Despite my newly found serenity, I decided to go back to the hospital after my sabbatical, wavering somewhat toward the end, but ready for one final push to the finish line.

A few months after I got back from Florida, I went to see a wonderful young lady named Allie, a patient with cystic fibrosis who had been waiting for a transplant for a few months. I had taken care of her for several years. She was highly intelligent and motivated to do well, and I liked her quite a bit.

Some of the other people on the team thought Allie was difficult because she was so diligent about her care—

compulsively adhering to her complicated medical regimen, always asking lots of questions about how she could take better care of herself, and sometimes challenging all of us to think of other ways to help her. When I saw her in clinic, I always planned on an hour, even for a routine appointment. After we went through her list of questions, she usually wanted to revisit a few items, just to make sure she fully understood the plan.

Allie had gotten increasingly sick and was now in full-blown respiratory failure, on a mechanical ventilator in the ICU. For two weeks, I visited her and her family a couple times a day in the ICU to talk about her condition. She was one of those patients who was so sick that, while she desperately needed a transplant, her tenuous status made the operation very risky. She was getting to the point where she might no longer be a candidate. The family knew it, and I knew it.

One morning, when I walked through the waiting room on my way into the ICU, I saw Allie's family and I knew right away that things had changed overnight. Her husband, Tony, had tears streaming down his face as he huddled with her parents.

I told them I'd be back as soon as I got a chance to check on Allie.

I felt my whole body tighten up as I went into her room. I said hello to the nurse, who gave me a quick update on Allie's condition: more difficult to oxygenate, lower blood pressure, high fever, the endotracheal tube down her throat suctioning out nasty green sputum. All signs that Allie's pneumonia was worsening, despite the wide array of antibiotics we were pumping into her.

As the nurse spoke to me, I scanned my surroundings, taking everything in: a sick young woman lying comatose in the bed; monitors displaying patient data that, if sustained, would be incompatible with life; the concerned nurse's hushed tones; the family in the waiting room, crying and holding each other. It was a familiar scenario. But today, in that moment, everything became silent. I closed my eyes.

The nurse continued talking, but I didn't hear her. The bedside monitors were shrieking, begging for attention I would not give them. I was being lulled into a trance by the sound of the ventilator blowing air in and out of my patient's lungs. Good air in, bad air out. Air that I had promised to change for this woman by giving her new lungs, just as I had for so many like her. But I wasn't going to get it done this time.

I needed to go tell Allie's family that she was not going to get a transplant, that she was going to die. But I didn't want to move. I wanted to stand there in the peace of my own quiet space, as if by not moving and not talking I could avoid facing the fact that we had failed Allie and her family. I wanted time to stop, or go backward to a time when she was well. A time when I was in better shape, too.

Finally, I heard the nurse say, "Dr. Weill? What do you think?" It was as though someone was talking to me underwater.

I opened my eyes and blinked against the sound of the monitors a few times, my sight a bit blurry, my thoughts unfocused. I shook my head a few times. "Thanks," I said. "I'll go talk to the family."

As I came to the double doors leading out of the ICU to the waiting room, I saw Tony and Allie's parents waiting for me in the hallway. I began speaking before the doors even shut behind me, wanting to get the words out as quickly as possible, as if I was giving Confession. "Umm...she's very sick." I stumbled for the words, even though I'd had this talk thousands of times in the past. I felt nauseated and looked around for a bathroom; there was one just a few feet away, right next to the waiting area. I prayed that no one was in it. *Hang on, David. Don't lose it.*

I thought back to one of the first times I was in the emergency room as a medical student at Charity Hospital in New Orleans. I was twenty-four. They wheeled in a gunshot victim, and I was the first to get to him. I pulled back the sheet and saw blood pouring out of multiple wounds in the guy's chest, including two right in the heart. I looked around for help and was relieved to see some senior residents running my way, grateful when they pushed me out of the way to attend to him.

This time, though, no one was coming to bail me out. I leaned against a wall to steady myself.

"She can't, I mean, we can't...she can't get a transplant," I mumbled. I was seeing spots and I felt suddenly overcome, at a loss for words. I grabbed Tony's forearm, less for his sake than for mine. I felt tears running down my face, and I reached into my pocket for a tissue. I didn't have one, so I used the sleeve of my sport coat. I was trying to compose myself and could see that the concern on the faces of her family was less for their daughter than for me.

Tony, this kind man who was about to lose his wife, put both arms around me, and I sobbed uncontrollably. Allie's mother handed me a tissue, as I apologized over and over for the mess I had become.

"It's okay, honey, we know how much you care about Allie," she said. "She really liked you and thought you were great."

I started shaking my head. *No, I'm not great. If I were, we wouldn't be having this fucking conversation.* I knew that wasn't true, but I couldn't keep the thoughts from coming. They flooded in and threatened to drown me. I was getting better, had found some new tools with which to navigate life—closeness to those that loved me, being more open with my emotions. But it was going to take a while. *For now, I have to accept the comfort from wherever it comes, even from the poor family of this dying patient.*

I told the family again—for what felt like the hundredth time—how sorry I was, and I went into the bathroom. I needed to get a hold of myself and clean up enough to walk through the hospital back to my office. I shut the door, took off my sport coat, and hung it on the door, noticing the trail of snot on the right-hand sleeve. I was still crying, but I'd slowed down a bit. I looked at myself in the mirror and saw who was staring back—a lost little boy with red eyes and a runny nose.

I stayed in the restroom for twenty minutes, until I thought I was together enough to make it back to my office. As I slowly walked the long hospital corridor, my head was down but my mind was sure.

I was done.

Thirty

Three months later

The first Monday of June 2016, I woke up before 5:00 a.m., staring straight ahead, stretching out my arms and legs one at a time, thinking about the day ahead.

But this day was going to be unlike any I'd had.

I had an email to send—it was time to get the decision off my chest that I'd made a few months earlier. It was an email that I wanted to send, but was reluctant to, given that it would mark the end of an important era of my professional life.

But before I got dressed to go to the hospital that day, I wanted to look through The Box.

I took out The Box from underneath the desk in my home office. It was a simple brown cardboard container, two feet high and a few feet wide. Nothing special about it on the outside—the magic was inside.

Inside that box was my transplant life.

The Box was filled with pictures and letters from my patients. There were thousands of them, which says more about the people I took care of than about me. I did my job, but they did the hard part, and then were gracious enough to write to me about it.

Over twenty-five years, they sent me stuff regularly—some scrawled on lined paper, some on fancy stationary embossed with their formal names, all of them handwritten. Some of the handwriting was shaky, like the writer was trying desperately to keep their hand still. It was probably due to a tremor—a side effect of one of the commonly used immunosuppression drugs, a side effect that neither they nor I could do anything about.

But they wrote anyway, and I read them all, usually more than once, as with a passage in a book that carried special meaning for me.

Many were simple thank-you notes, like you would write to the host after a dinner party. But the content was different. Instead of reading, "Thanks for the good company and good food. We'll have you all over soon," these read, "You saved my life. I can't thank you enough," "You gave me my daughter back," and "Your team was tremendous—my family thanks you." The notes were at the very least uplifting and validating. And on some days, the words downright floored me.

"We pray for you every day."

When I was working in the hospital all the time, I loved getting those letters, and now they're the script that runs through my head when I sit in the quiet of my home office and think back on those years.

But I received other kinds of notes also—from families of patients we'd transplanted and lost. Those said things like, "I know you did the best you could—thank you for your efforts. We think about him every day. And you," and

"I hope you and your team can learn something from the death of our mother." These letters were the most profound—combinations of the kind of grace and grief that's unfathomable to those who've never experienced it. Those hit me the hardest. Those are the ones I reread the most.

Some letters contained pictures—Christmas cards and shots of patients being active and enjoying life: a thumbs-up from a double lung recipient on a golf course in Hawaii; a mother with her three kids on a ski mountain, holding their ski poles above their heads; a mountain climber on top of Mount Rainier with a sign that reads, "Lung Transplant: 10/14/2007."

There was a picture of two of my patients holding hands while skydiving. I'm not sure what about getting a transplant made them want to jump out of an airplane, but I had a surprising number of patients tell me after a transplant that they wanted to do it. All I asked of them was that they not tell me *when* they were going to do it—I didn't need the additional worry. I had enough trouble getting—and keeping—my own parachute open at times.

And finally, there was a picture from a cliffside overlooking the Pacific—a wedding party applauding a couple's first kiss as man and wife, the beautiful bride a transplant patient in her mid-twenties. The scene looked straight out of a magazine. On this day I held the picture for a few minutes, looking at the happy faces, thinking about what she did, and then, immodestly, about what I'd done.

I sifted through The Box some more, rain and fog enveloping my office, the soft thunder a soundtrack to my career retrospective. I reread some of my favorites, the greatest hits.

I smiled and shook my head, turning the cards over and over in my hands. *How lucky I have been.*

I stayed absorbed by the contents of The Box until an hour had passed and it was time to go. I closed it and slid it back under my desk, where it would sit until the next time I needed it.

I showered, shaved, and went into my walk-in closet to get dressed. What do you wear on the day you're going to resign? Something nice, like dress pants and a blazer? Or jeans and an old ratty T-shirt? Clothes that scream, "I'm done!"

I decided to split the difference and go with jeans, a blue button-down shirt, and a dark green sport coat.

As I sat down to put on my shoes, Ava walked into the closet on her tiptoes. She shared my affliction of waking up early and rarely slept past 6:00 a.m.—much to her mother's consternation. She handed me my shoes.

"Where are you going?"

"To a meeting." I got down on my knees, so my face was level with hers. "Do you want to skip school and come with me?"

Her eyes brightened. "YEAH!"

I shook my head. "You know you can't do that."

She laughed. "I know, but I want to."

I was glad she was oblivious to all that was going on. She had a whole life ahead of her to deal with this kind of shit. I also thought of my dad, and all the mornings I spent in his closet watching him get dressed when I was little. I was grateful he wasn't alive to watch me going through this. But I know he would have wanted me to go into the hospital that day with my head held high, proud of what I had accomplished in the last twenty years.

I squeezed Ava tightly.

"Do you want some bacon, Daddy? I'm making some for me."

This was a common ritual between the two of us before anyone else was awake. She would make six pieces of bacon: five for her, one for me.

"No, none for me, thanks, sweetheart. I've got to go soon. But you can get me a glass of wine." I looked at her, stone-faced, giving her no sense that I was kidding.

She didn't smile either, not sure if I was serious. She looked at me and said, "For *breakfast?*"

I shrugged my shoulders as if to say, "Why not?" She shrugged.

"Just kidding," I finally said. *But maybe I wasn't.* "Got to go, I'll see you later."

Hit send. No, not yet.

I wanted to reread the email one last time.

"I am writing to let you know that I'll be leaving Stanford effective July 1…Everyone needs a new challenge from time to time, and I am very excited to enter this new phase of my life and for the experiences that lie ahead for my family and me."

"Thank you for your hard work over the years. Our efforts at providing excellence on behalf of the very sick people who count on us have always been paramount. Nothing should get in the way of this vital mission."

Send.

Then I waited. But for what? Responses from the 150 people I'd copied? Calls from my closest colleagues? Or for my regret to set in, causing me to scramble to compose another email saying the previous one was a mistake, a rash misjudgment, an April Fool's joke—in June?

I then heard the steady chime of incoming emails.

I spent the next few hours reading the incoming messages. Some expressed surprise, but many didn't. My angst at work over the past couple of years, especially after my father died, had been fairly obvious. The emails varied in tone and substance but were mostly eloquent and touching. My colleagues thanked me for the patients I had helped and for my leadership of the team. Even some of the people in the hospital with whom I had clashed sent gracious emails expressing their gratitude for my efforts, reminding me that I needed to do better with the people with whom I disagreed. *I was trying, though, and that represented progress.*

I also posted the email on my Facebook page, so my friends and patients would know. The responses were mostly congratulatory—some were incredulous ("Retiring?! How old are you?" and "Now what are you going to do?")—but all indicated that they appreciated my efforts. People seemed to sense that I'd given it my all and that it had taken a chunk out of me—a sacrifice worth making but, like all sacrifices, one that had come at a personal cost.

As I sat in my office that day, I wasn't at all down. I didn't want the job anymore, didn't want that life anymore. I told myself to concentrate on the end result. I didn't want to be there anymore, and on that point, some of my superiors were in vehement agreement, making it clear to me that they were more than eager to bring in a new leader of the program. During my time on sabbatical, the hospital leadership concluded that the program could survive without me, and I came to understand that I could live without it.

I had come to the point where I had to leave—not because of the job, but because of how I did my job. Too much pushing against other people and too much pushing myself to save all the patients, all the time. It had worn out the people I worked for. And it had worn me out.

I sat there, staring out the window, thinking about what I might do next. Not for the rest of my life, but for the next few hours. The sun was streaming in, not a cloud in the sky. I smiled slightly. I thought about how much, if I left California for good, I would miss days like this.

And a career like this.

My career thus far had given me everything. It beat me to pieces, fulfilled me, and gave me a daily purpose—and had demanded a lot in return. But I couldn't have asked for anything more. I worked hard, committed myself to what I believed in, and helped a lot of people during the most precarious moments of their lives.

Later, when the leaders at Stanford asked me if I wanted a farewell reception, I declined. In those email messages, I had all I could ask for.

And as I sat there, I thought, *I did my best,* which, sadly, was probably the first time in my life that I'd really ever felt that way. This time, in that office, on that day, I thought it and, more importantly, I believed it.

Transplant made me who I was—I would never be the same given what I had experienced. And I didn't want to be.

PART THREE

The doctor is effective only when he himself is affected. Only the wounded physician heals.
—Carl Jung

One

2016
New Orleans, Louisiana

I always figured I'd come back to New Orleans one way or the other, either in a box, to be buried above ground, as the locals say, or under better, more hopeful circumstances. But there was a paradox to my return: for most, New Orleans is a place you go to lose your shit, not to get your shit together. Nonetheless, here I was.

For the first time in our lives, Jackie and I decided to move not for a new job, a new hospital, or a chance to renovate a transplant program, but for a better reason: to make a new life.

Before leaving Stanford, I'd looked at a couple of jobs that were similar to all the others I'd had in the past: a broken transplant program to fix, a chance to build something better, a problem to solve. Jackie and I went to the recruiting dinners, met with some impressive people, and heard their pitches about how I was just what their hospital needed.

We decided to turn them all down, not with any sense of disappointment, but rather a feeling of relief. We chose not to jump right back in, instead recognizing the need to take time to regroup, for me to heal emotionally, to put our focus where it belonged: on each other and our daughters. We decided this together—indicative of an evolution in our relationship that would not have been possible when I was on my career trajectory. We evolved because I evolved.

New Orleans was the setting we picked for this new way of life. Because of the sense of comfort it provided, because my mother and sister Leslie were there, because of the life-long friends I wanted to reconnect with. It might surprise those who have visited the city as tourists, but to me, New Orleans offered a warm feeling of familiarity as well as, ironically, given its reputation, sanity and stability when I most needed it.

We moved in time to enroll the kids at Isidore Newman School, the same school I had attended. Moving home in the August heat and humidity was not ideal, but it was a clear reminder each time I walked out the door that I was not in California anymore, which would turn out to be but one of the many contrasts between my old and new life. Acclimating to the stickiness of the air was a relatively minor adjustment. A more significant transition involved having—for the first time ever—no real structure to my day: no patients to keep me focused, people to manage, or transplant program to run.

I started most mornings with a walk in Audubon Park with my sister Leslie along an oak-lined trail. On one end of the park sat Tulane University and Holy Name of Jesus Church and, on the other end, the Mississippi River. The park is home to thousands of ducks, egrets, and herons that, along with the church bells, provided a soothing soundtrack. It was a good, slow way to start my mornings, quite different from the early hustle to the hospital that had been my routine for so long. The rest of the day I puttered in my home office, trying to stay out of Jackie's hair, so as not to disrupt the rhythm she'd developed all those years while I was at the hospital.

After a few weeks of roaming around the house, I decided to rent an office in a busy commercial corridor uptown. The space was on the second floor of an old building, above a hair salon. The office took up an entire floor, far more than I needed, and had an open floor plan, only partially divided by glass partitions. I moved all my father's home office furniture into my new office. After he died, it had been collecting dust in an empty office at Leslie's law firm. Now I had his desk, computer table, and leather couch, which I had sat on many times as a young boy. Some of those times were when my father wanted to have a serious conversation, and others we were just hashing out the issues of the day on a weekend afternoon.

I put a sign Jackie had made on the door that read "Weill Consulting Group." A name that lacked some imagination but seemed appropriate for a business that lacked, at least initially, any specific mission. I also decided to hire an assistant. I was a little vague on why I needed one, my only rationale that most real businesses had one. Through contacts, I found a pleasant woman named Pam whose husband of many years had recently died and who had also just moved back to New Orleans after a long time away. When I hired her, the job description was unclear, but I knew we needed a phone, an internet connection, and a couple of computers. She set these up within a couple of hours on her first day.

I had business cards made and hired someone to work on a website that featured my experience as a transplant doctor. Once that was done, I sat on my father's couch and waited, sometimes reading one of the transplant journals I'd stacked on the coffee table; other times, I sent out a few emails to colleagues in the transplant field, letting them know where I was and what I was doing.

On the second Monday of our new business, Pam and I were sitting in our office when the phone rang. The office was big enough that, despite the open space, I couldn't see her at her desk. But I could hear her. "Weill Consulting Group, this is Pam." It all sounded so professional, so official. I stood up and walked to the back of the office where she sat. I heard her hang up the phone.

"Who was it?" I asked.

"Wrong number." Deflated, I walked back to the couch.

Later that day, Pam made her way to my side of the office and said, "David?"

I was lying on the couch and had apparently fallen asleep while reading about the newest technology in detecting lung transplant rejection. I sat up abruptly, wiping the drool from my cheek. "Yes?"

"Sorry to wake you, but I'm going to go ahead and go."

"Oh, okay. Thanks. See you tomorrow," I said, still in a fog.

Pam looked at me, surveying the scene. My hair was sticking straight up, wrinkled T-shirt, reading glasses on top of the medical journal next to the couch. "Do you need anything?"

"No," I forced a smile, "I'm good." I heard her leave out the front door. I lay back down. I stared at the high ceiling, running my eyes along a crack in the white paint. I could hear the techno beat and loud chatter from the hair salon. I thought about how I got here. *What am I going to do every day?* I let my thoughts wander. *I should be racing around a hospital somewhere, large and in charge, trying to make sick people better. Instead I'm hanging out above a hair salon.*

But I quickly stopped myself from going down that rabbit hole, saying out loud, 'Slowly. Slowly."

Two

"**A**re you still a doctor?"

I was at the gym on an especially sticky August morning when I ran into an old high school friend trying to address the midlife spread. I was on a citywide gym tour, trying out places I might want to join. He came up to me while I was doing bicep curls—not a time I usually want to engage in conversation of any kind, much less this one.

Are you still a doctor? He probably was being sincere. Still, I could feel the blood going to my face, in my past an early warning that what was coming would not be good. Even now, my response could have been—maybe should have been, "Are you still a fuckhead?" Just a few years earlier, I would have seriously considered cocking back one of the dumbbells in my hands and smashing it into his skull, eliminating questions of this sort altogether.

Instead, I just gave a fake smile. "I guess once a doctor, always a doctor," I said, which avoided my having to tell the whole story of how I had gotten to this point. I was happy when he moved on to easier topics, the banal questions old friends ask: "How's your new house?" "How do Jackie and the kids like New Orleans?" "Where have you been going

302

out to eat?" Safe conversation as we stood among the free weights and treadmills.

Are you still a doctor? The question stayed with me for the rest of the day. The seemingly innocent question had irritated a nerve that I had exposed when I left Stanford. Having been re-introduced to people I hadn't seen in the twenty-six years I'd been gone from New Orleans, I was now getting a steady stream of similar questions, one version after the other.

Or worse, I imagined the gossip among my peer group of middle-aged professional men: "You remember David? He's retired now."

At first, I corrected anyone who made that assumption, to set the record straight. "No, just wanted a change of direction," or "Wanted to spend more time with my family," or the easy out, "I was ready to get back home."

Lately, I had been just letting the retirement comment go. People said it, I was guessing, merely out of interest, or perhaps amazement, given that I was only fifty-two, at least in calendar years. Some probably even thought retirement—whatever it is—was a desirable goal, one you spend a lifetime trying to achieve, clawing your way to a "magic number." I knew one thing for certain: I was not finished with my career, and I saw this phase—if that's even what it was—as the next chapter in a book whose ending was a mystery to me.

But the question of what was next for me was legitimate, one that I thought about nearly all the time, especially when I was first back in New Orleans, which was only just a couple of months after a long period—some might say too long—of having been *very much* a doctor.

Three

Soon after we moved back, I was standing at a cocktail party in the Garden District. I looked for someone I wanted to talk to when Taylor, my girlfriend during high school and college, walked up to me.

"Hey," she said in her soft Southern lilt. We hugged and began the awkward conversation of high school sweethearts when they've reached middle age. "How are Jackie and the kids?" "Are you enjoying being back in New Orleans?" "Who have you seen since you've been back?"

"So what are you up to these days?" she asked. My least favorite subject.

"Not much…trying to find a drink." She laughed. "Not right this second. I mean generally." She took a swig from her glass. I waited for the conversation to move on. It didn't.

"So, you had enough of all that doctoring stuff?" she smiled.

I shrugged and gave a fake half-smile—searching for one of my throwaway lines. "Just wanted to take a break, be back home."

She nodded, seeming to assume there was more to it. When you've known each other for thirty-five years, it's hard to hide behind a bullshit line like that.

The smile left her face. "Yeah, I get that, David, but had you had *enough*?"

As I lay in bed later that night, replaying the party and the conversation with Taylor, I thought about the word she'd used. *Enough.*

What a dumbass word for someone like me to hear. I'd been hearing it all my life. From my father: "Haven't you moved *enough*?" "How much money is *enough*?" From others: "Haven't you ridden your bike *enough*?" From those closest to me: "Haven't you worked *enough*? Chased your career *enough*?"

Shouldn't we know when enough is enough?

Well sure, ideally.

But does an alcoholic—with sparkling ice cubes and a fine twist of lime in a glass with gin and tonic placed at eye level on a bar top—know when enough is enough? A coke fiend, with a thin white line teed up right in front of him? It is, as far as I'm concerned, heroic if any of these people find the strength, or perhaps clarity of thought, to say, "No, thanks. I'm good, I've had *enough*."

I used to think the concept of "enough" was for losers.

Enough. I couldn't even spell it. Until I had had enough.

Four

During my last year in Palo Alto, I had been seeing Stephanie Brown, the therapist and author. I had read her book *Speed* many times, highlighting sections I liked and writing notes in the margins. Much of what we talked about in our sessions centered around the concepts in her book—that going fast in life was merely a way to distract ourselves from the deep emotions that are fundamental to a contemplative, connected life. Her thesis, which I had found particularly helpful, was that speed, disguised as ambition and achievement, or even simple multitasking, was really just a way to avoid deep intimacy—a relationship with ourselves and with others.

Over a year, meeting sometimes once a week but often twice, we made progress—or, to be more accurate, I gained insight into why I did the things I did. Therapy, as for most people, became a way for me to say to another person what I subconsciously already knew. I formed the words in my brain, which was one form of learning, and then heard myself say them out loud, which is another form of learning.

And for Stephanie's help, I had been grateful.

Since I'd moved away, I wanted to find another therapist to continue the work I had started in California. Rather than find one in New Orleans, which is small enough that your therapist is likely to know everyone in your family and circle of friends, and likely to have remembered you from high school. Instead I chose a therapist in Los Angeles named Michael who would meet with me every week via videoconference.

"Post-traumatic stress disorder."

I searched Michael's face on the computer screen, thinking about these words, the books I had read, the sympathy I had felt for its victims. He and I had been meeting for a few months, and I had become accustomed to speaking intimately with him in this virtual format.

"As in PTSD, the thing the soldiers get?" I asked.

"Yep. Same thing," he said. He did not elaborate. He was going to let this sink in. It felt like an hour, the silence seeming particularly loud.

I slowly began to speak, thinking out loud. "What would my trauma be? I don't remember being shot at. Although there might have been a few people at Stanford who considered it." I laughed too heartily. Michael wasn't laughing. "How could I have PTSD?"

"You think you don't deserve to have it?"

"That sounds like something a therapist would say." Now Michael smiled and shrugged. "Well, do you?"

"Do I what?" I was stalling. I looked at the clock. Still twenty minutes left in our session. *This might be a good time to "lose" the connection.*

"Deserve to have PTSD. You watched a lot of people die—young people. People whom you thought you should have saved."

I shifted in my chair, looked away from the screen, and stiffened. "I did." Now a bit more indignant and defensive. "But it wasn't like I was walking around worried about which villager might be hiding an AK-47. Or driving around in a Humvee trying to avoid the next roadside bomb."

"True. But you experienced real trauma. People died. Patients for whom you felt responsible."

I looked at him, my lips pursed. Then the tears came, slowly at first, and then pouring out like a waterfall.

"Yep." I stopped to blow my nose. I took a deep breath.

Michael waited. "Do you blame yourself for those people dying?"

"Yeah, part of me does."

"How does that make you feel?"

I laughed out loud. "Now that's a therapist question for sure. Next are you going to ask me how I feel about my mother?"

He looked straight at me, expressionless. "How does it make you feel?"

"How does it look like it makes me feel? Like shit."

He nodded. "But does it seem reasonable? That you can control who lives and who dies? You're a religious guy. Does that make sense?"

"No. But that doesn't mean I don't think it. Or did think it."

He paused for a moment. "Can I ask you to question that thought?"

I shrugged my shoulders. "You can ask."

Neither of us said anything for few moments. I wiped my nose again. Then it was time to wrap up the session.

When I disconnected from the call, I looked around my empty office. Post-traumatic stress disorder. Really? Was my trauma that significant? I was unconvinced. I would need to process this. Slowly.

Five

Spring 2018

A carefully crafted career—the right grades in college, the grind in medical school, the best residencies. The strategic career moves, climbing the ladder. The sacrifices I had made, all the sacrifices my wife and kids had made. All ending in a slow burn rather than a fiery crash. Burnout was an easy label, but it was more complicated than that. I needed more information to figure out what had really happened.

Where would I go to find it? Ironically, I was headed back to Stanford. I had enrolled in an executive education course called the *Innovative Health Care Leader* because of the session entitled "The High Cost of Physician Burnout."

I showed up on the campus of the Stanford Business School campus on a typically beautiful May morning. It was less than two years since I had left, and this was my first time back on campus. Leading the seminar on burnout was one of the country's leading experts on the subject, Dr. Tait Shanafelt, whom Stanford had recently hired to lead a new program directed at physician wellness—the first of its kind to be offered at an academic medical center. The medical school had hired Dr. Shanafelt, I learned while sitting in his session, as part of the dean's office and given him an endowed chair, which I thought reflected just how significant the problem was. *How enlightened*, I thought. *It just came a few years too late for me.*

The session comprised about fifty healthcare leaders from around the country: CEOs of hospitals, executives in the pharmaceutical industry, and leaders of academic medical centers. I sat in the class, listening to the description of physician burnout, why it happens, who is most likely to "contract" it. He described all the symptoms I had when I had left Stanford: insomnia, irritability, lack of engagement with my colleagues. At five foot ten, I weighed only 137 pounds, and it had been increasingly difficult to explain my weight loss as purely a side effect of cycling. As I sat there listening to the symptoms, I thought of how by the end of my time at Stanford I'd felt burned to a crisp. How accurately he was describing my symptoms! I had known something was wrong, but until now I didn't have a name for it. When the symptoms developed, my first reaction was to scold myself—*Get your act together, get tougher, get going*—rather than seek help. I was channeling the voices from my residency mentors, my coaches, and my Dad.

I found myself looking around to see if I was the only one nodding their head in agreement as Dr. Shanafelt went through slide after slide that detailed the findings of his research. No one else seemed to register a response. I wasn't surprised. We in the medical field have excellent poker faces, developed over years of training and patient care experience, a mask that is every bit as important a tool as our stethoscope or scalpel.

Dr. Shanafelt ticked through study after study indicating that physicians are burning out at an alarming rate, which is bad not only for the doctors it affects, but especially for the patients they are treating.

Toward the end of my time at Stanford, I'd carried around the image of myself as being so burnt beyond recognition that you could only identify me by my dental records. And I didn't even realize it had a name, didn't even know it was a common phenomenon. *I blew my own diagnosis.*

I continued to read about it more and more. One day I sat in my office for an entire day and read through all the research I could find in the medical literature. I learned that the rate of burnout is higher among physicians than any other occupation, due to concrete aspects of the job: the electronic medical records, the bureaucracy and lack of control, the declining status of physicians in the culture.

However, in my reading about "physician wellness," which certainly sounds better than "burnout"—less dramatic, more clinical, a sanitized way to say a doctor has lost his or her way—I couldn't relate to much of what was driving the high incidence of physicians who were affected. Nowhere in the research I read, or in conversations with the experts I would eventually seek out, was there discussion of something obvious that seemed to me fundamental: These doctors were tired of seeing patients die, and in failing to save them, they—that is, I—had lost a healthy sense of emotional detachment, and instead came to see each new patient as a personal test of his or her own self-worth. And in a specialty like mine, in which the survival rates were tenuous at best, this was a self-perpetuating cycle, a downward spiral.

Six

My professional plan—which had started out as vague in those early days but was gradually coming into focus—was to assist transplant programs across the country that were in need of help, that were confronting the same struggles I had faced in my own career.

As the months went on, I consulted for transplant programs facing a variety of challenges, as well as hospitals that were seeking to create a new transplant program.

I couldn't very well take out an ad to the effect of: "Have a struggling transplant program? Call David and set your worries free." I knew only too well that hospitals, particularly those with an underperforming program, are circumspect, seeking strict confidentiality. This was something I respected entirely. Ultimately, I didn't need do anything to attract business—clients just came by word of mouth. Soon the work was really starting to pick up.

The process of consulting work intrigued me. I would look at reams of outcome data before I arrived on-site. Once at the hospital, I arranged interviews with essentially everyone involved with the transplant programs, from the CEO of the hospital to the physicians to the nurses and dieticians. I have often thought I should also interview the staff who clean the patient rooms, given how much they probably know about what really goes on. I am essentially like an investigative reporter who shows up to learn what really happened—the backstory about why a program is underperforming.

I continue to be amazed by the information people are willing to disclose in my interviews. Team members tend to start out being cautious, but over the course of our conversation, I am often able to draw out of them fairly easily what the primary issues are. I find that most people are genuine in their desire for the problem to be solved, and if that means telling me some dirt, they're eager to do it.

One subset of transplant consulting that quickly became my specialty was transplant programs that were dysfunctional because of poor interpersonal relationships among the transplant team. Ironic, huh?

But the more I thought about it, the more I thought that hiring me to negotiate a détente made sense—perhaps similar in some ways to how former generals are often used to negotiate peace. Because they've seen war firsthand—and personally felt the toll of losing soldiers on the battlefield— they will work relentlessly to find ways to avoid it. When I observe it now as a consultant, the in-fighting within a team strikes me clearly as a counterproductive behavior. In fact, thinking back on my own participation in similar skirmishes now makes me cringe. From the benefit of my vantage point now, one step removed, the fighting seems a complete waste of energy and time—especially considering the stakes involved in what a transplant team is trying to get accomplished.

But due to everything I had seen, had lived, I am proud that I have been able to help make other programs better, help them to identify and implement tangible improvements. Things have become so busy that, rather than working with one program at a time, as in the beginning, I now work with as many as reach out to me, often simultaneously. It's now my job to tell transplant programs some uncomfortable truths, truths that—despite the fact that I'm being paid to deliver them—the leadership sometimes does not want to hear.

I found my purpose, though. It's simple, actually: to help the programs work more effectively so they can help people. In that way, I'm still indirectly helping patients. It works for me, and it works for my clients, whom I think of as partners. It has been a satisfying way for me to contribute, to apply what I know. *This is progress.*

I also received calls now and then about the same type of job I had at Stanford: leading a transplant program and developing a multidisciplinary center for patients with end-stage lung diseases. I listened to what these potential employers had to say, and I must admit, these discussions stirred up my passion to tackle a new project.

Most of the hospitals had transplant programs that were struggling and, although in the past I would have jumped at the opportunity to renovate another program, I found the timing just wasn't right. I was settling into my new life, and more important, Jackie was settling into our new life, having lunch with friends she quickly made, working on our house, making it a home for our family, something she did with great skill and careful attention. She was done with the old life, and she had a right to be. I owed it to her to give this new life a chance—a life outside the hospital, that was free of late-night donor calls, my worry, and preoccupation.

As I turned these jobs down, it seemed hard for some of the "suitors" to believe I was done with this type of work. One chief medical officer from a large hospital in Texas put it more bluntly when he was interviewing me.

"How old are you? This seems like the career choice of someone who has just become lazy."

A year or two out of the game had given me some healthy detachment. I laughed the comment off—something I certainly wouldn't have been able to do even a few years prior.

"I'm learning to help in a different way now."

"Hell. I don't blame you," he said, to my surprise. "I'd do it, too, if I could."

I got a lot of that from people I talked to who were "still in the game." It's a tough world, and I suspect there are more transplant people than I would have thought who are suffering from the demands of the culture and looking for an exit ramp. This concerns me, because of how desperately I know we need good, dedicated people in the trenches. The hospital in Texas where the skeptic had interrogated me ultimately did become a client of mine, and we eventually made substantial progress in getting their transplant program back on track.

Win-win.

Seven

Summer 2018

The author Andre Dubus III supposedly once said that a memoir is not about "what happened," but about "what the fuck happened." That resonated with me. I've tried to keep this in mind, to articulate what really transpired, carefully and honestly.

At the end of this chapter in my life, as I move forward toward the next one, I find myself asking: What did all this mean? One conclusion I reached soon after leaving California was that I needed to leave the hospital, to stop, not only for my own good but for the good of my patients. It certainly was not that I no longer cared. Quite the opposite—I cared about the patients so much that I didn't want them to have to be cared for by someone who was working out some of his own issues. In retrospect I would have wanted, like most people, to walk away on my own terms, make an elegant farewell while I was still fit both physically and emotionally. Instead, I feel that I was compelled to limp away, wounds still bleeding, but scared to give it up because I didn't know what came next. *Who would I be without the job?*

My fear had been that I would be the doctor equivalent of former NFL quarterback Brett Favre—riding a tractor mower, drinking a beer, wondering if I should give it one last shot. Obviously, medicine would be fine without me, but would I be fine without medicine? How would I meet my needs for gratitude without the daily scorecard of which patients I had "managed to keep alive"? In essence, how would I know for sure that I was worthwhile?

What eventually saved me? The reflection, the meaningful consulting work with transplant programs, the writing, the family, the therapy, the slowing down.

And this is what I came to understand during those long walks around Audubon Park: Transplant medicine had been my perfect vehicle. It was a means of expression, giving me everything I craved: gratitude, glory, competition, even pain. A way to feel love from other people, to have people tell me that I'd saved them. And for them to mean it. A way to ride in on a white horse to save the day and rescue everyone, whether I'd just met them, as was most often the case, or whether it was someone close to me: my father.

There was a downside to all this, I came to find out—to the high I felt in giving people hope. A referendum each day on your self-worth, based on who got better and who didn't, wasn't just foolish—especially in my field—it led to what felt like a train crash happening in slow motion. With lots of painstaking work and good fortune, I was able to recover from it. For that, I thank God every day.

You might think that, because of the hurt I felt, I would be resentful about the field of transplant medicine, as if that could be rational. But I'm not. In fact, quite the opposite. Transplant was my religion before I had any. I worshipped faithfully, and I thought that to be devout was to be saintly, and that through my devotion I could save every patient. This was before I realized I wasn't saving anyone by myself. God was—or whatever spiritual force you believe in. And when I finally realized that, I knew I was going to be okay.

Eight

During the first twelve months I was back in New Orleans I was focused on understanding, on healing, on picking up the pieces. And now, well into the second twelve months, I was being tested on how far I had come. Two people with whom I was close died unexpectedly, and the grief resulting from the two deaths shook me hard.

The first was someone who was like an older brother. Gene Lafitte died suddenly of a brain aneurysm while at dinner. One day I was talking with him about football, and the next day he was gone. I comforted his family, who were like my second family. And then I took care of myself, sitting in the bathtub in the morning, crying at times, and laughing to myself at others while remembering some of the funny conversations that we'd had. It felt like a normal response to death, much different than when my father died, when I'd had trouble conjuring up any emotion at all.

The second was the death of my twenty-one-year-old niece, Katy, a devastating tragedy for our family. This evoked the full a range of emotions of which humans are capable: pain, loss, anger at the victim, and mostly a heavy dose of hopelessness—the sort my daughters would experience for the first time but, as I told them, not the last. Some would say later, whether at Katy's service, by email or text, or in the park, that hers was a senseless death. In response to which I found myself thinking, *Does it matter? Senseless or not, death is death. Gone is gone.*

Nothing I could say could help my sister and brother-in-law with the devastation they felt. There was no use in providing doctorly words of sympathy or attempting to express empathy. The truth was I had no idea what they must have felt, so why pretend?

But I was the one who told my mother, my dear mother. I went to the apartment to which she had moved after my father died, so I could tell her face to face and be there with her, for another family loss. I remember the look on her face, the pain of realizing that one of her grandchildren was gone forever. Seeing my mother, on that day, in that way, made me desperate to go find my own kids and hug them until they said, "Dad, it's okay. You can let go. We're not going anywhere."

Yet there were no guarantees of that—for my children or anyone else's. My work certainly taught me that, and as of late, my personal life was full of fresh reminders that death follows us everywhere—the hospital, sure, but also elsewhere. It follows everyone. When it happens—if you're healthy—you cry, you grieve, you take time to remember. Then you dust yourself off and move on, wounded but alive.

Nine

Fall 2018

Still in bed on an early October morning, I looked out our bedroom window, watching the water from a lazy drizzle run slowly down the pane. Being away for so long, I had forgotten how subtle fall was in New Orleans, a nearly imperceptible lifting of the smothering heat and humidity, as though someone had ever so slightly turned down the steam bath.

Today I wouldn't be talking with a sick patient about getting a transplant, or giving out bad news to a family meeting in a room just outside the ICU. Last night there had been no phone call about a set of lungs, no hearing about some anonymous donor's tragedy, no decision to make about whether one of my patients should get a transplant that night. Without all of this, I had slept for nine hours for the first time in memory.

I thought about my schedule for the day. First, walk the dog around the park. For two years now, I had been smiling and nodding at the same people I passed, those who, I assumed, had regular jobs and regular lives. Then I would swim some laps, finding a cool and quiet underwater sanctuary. I preferred swimming to cycling now—no hills to climb, nothing to conquer.

But I would wonder.

Would this be one of those days when I wished with all my heart that I was out of bed early, rushing to work, and stomping through the hospital, pupils dilated, hair on fire?

Maybe. There would be days that I thought about this question, I was certain.

I'd be lying if I said I didn't miss some aspects of my life in California. The natural beauty, the innovative culture, and mostly my cycling buddies—lifelong friends I'd enjoyed meeting for a beer and conversation. But most days, I didn't miss my work in the hospital there. I'd found a new way to contribute, to make things better for patients, without making things worse for myself.

I thought about something I'd read the day before, that the first twenty years of one's life is when genius can happen, and the rest is all reflection. During the period this book covers, I had reached twenty years of my life in transplant medicine. I guess I'm now in the reflection stage.

What I find I am thinking about now is what a privilege it was to do what I did and still have the time to reflect upon it all, from this new vantage point—all before breakfast. To see what I've seen, to do what I've done, to bear witness to my patients' courage. It's not only humbling; it has been the experience of a lifetime.

I may never again go through anything quite like my time in California—and hope I never let things get so out of balance again. But I wouldn't trade it for anything. I have come to see that I had to leave behind one version of my life, of my identity, for there to be an opportunity to create a better one. How could I not be grateful for that?

I've moved on and, from what I've heard, my former colleagues at Stanford have as well. I've gained the long view of transplant programs and how they go through a series of progressions that reflects the history of our own civilization—some an improvement, some a regression from the one before. It was natural for a new civilization to emerge at Stanford. This is healthy for transplant programs, for companies, for most institutions.

I do take great pride and satisfaction in knowing my work and our team rehabilitated a struggling program and changed the lives of hundreds of patients. Despite the challenges along the way, we did it successfully for eleven years, achieving some of the best outcomes in the country and, importantly, avoiding the unwanted attention of external agencies charged with ensuring transplant program quality. Eleven years is a long time in our field. But it was time for a new perspective, a new leader, an unjaded point of view.

Stanford hired new surgeons, as I thought was needed all along. Some of the nurses I worked with still call me periodically to see how I'm doing—and to complain a little. I don't have much contact with anyone else there, but I wish them well. I'm proud of what I helped to build, since a well-performing program helps patients, with or without me.

I was now focused more on the sounds in the park— the ducks whistling, dozens of them, their high-pitched squeals traveling across the lake, through the oak trees, and into our bedroom. I've learned that the ducks migrate here in November. From what the locals tell me, they leave in March. But I won't be.

I was home now and happy.

That was also the year—the first since my father had died, that I forgot the anniversary of his death. November 6 came and went without notice, without a single thought of him. When I realized weeks later that I had forgotten, I wondered, *Does this mean I'm moving on in a healthy way, or that I'm an uncaring asshole?* My new self decided there may not be a profound explanation. I just forgot and had moved to another stage of my grieving process—a stage where I was able to focus on what was right in front of me, while still remembering all of what came before.

In November of 2018, two years since I'd left Stanford, I was flying back from London after consulting with a company developing a drug to treat chronic rejection of lungs in transplant patients. This was an exciting part of the new way I interacted with my field, which has not only been my life's work, but in many ways was my first true love, before I met Jackie, before Hannah and Ava were born.

Toward the end of the flight, the flight attendant came around to pass out the landing cards for Customs for our arrival. I took out my reading glasses and a pen. Name, date of birth, passport number. Then I came to the part that asked for my occupation. I smiled to myself.

Are you still a doctor? I didn't hesitate. I wrote "Physician." *Then. Now.*

Epilogue

Winter 2019

I woke up early one January morning. I could hear the rain on the roof above our bedroom and the thunder rumbling. I was wide awake from the moment I opened my eyes.

I got up and dressed, donning my hospital uniform: jeans, a white button-down shirt, a navy blazer. As I came downstairs to our kitchen, Jackie was helping the kids get ready to leave for school. The kids were cramming food into their mouths while checking their phones.

Before Hannah left to drive her sister to school, she looked up from her phone for an instant and looked me over.

"Dad." She reached out and ran her hand over my sport coat. "What are you doing? Why are you so dressed up?" She had seen me mainly in shorts and a T-shirt over the last couple of years.

"Going to the hospital. To see patients. You remember when I used to do that?" I smiled.

She shrugged. "Not really," and went back to her phone.

"Not really?" I guess she missed all that. Okay...

Once the kids left, I sat at the kitchen table with Jackie while she drank her coffee. We would take this quiet part of the morning, after the kids went off to school and before she left for the gym, to catch up. We looked at each other for a few moments.

"When are you going to be done with this?" She asked the question knowingly, but without antagonism. It was a question with so much backstory.

"Done with what?" I asked. She smiled. "That's a complicated question," I said. No further words were necessary for a couple who had been through what we had.

I was joining the transplant team part time at Ochsner Medical Center, a large tertiary care center just a few miles from our house. Some of the doctors I had trained at Stanford now worked there, and I would be providing, in a small way, assistance both in the outpatient setting and with program management. The hospital leadership had been asking since I moved back if I was interested in helping out and was willing to accommodate my request to take a small first step. The prospect of working with people I already knew, whom I also liked and respected, felt right, as did serving my hometown transplant center.

I was to attend an orientation session that morning, and by the afternoon, I would see my first patients in well over two years.

The orientation was held in a large conference room. Outside was a sign that read, "Orientation for New Physicians." Inside there were tables set up, with our names on small cardboard signs. I looked at all the names, searching for my seat. Jane Flanders, Advanced Practice Provider. Christian Ellis, Urology. Steve Schmidt, Podiatry. *There it was.* David Weill, Pulmonary Transplant.

The person running the orientation, a cheerful woman from the medical staff office, introduced herself.

"You must be one of the new physicians." She extended her hand.

"Yes." She took my hand and covered it with both of hers.

"And where did you do your residency?" *I haven't been asked that in a long time.* Then it occurred to me: *She thinks I only just finished my residency.* I didn't know whether to be flattered, because she thought I looked young enough to be newly trained, or insulted that she didn't know who I was. I chose the former.

"Oh, I finished my residency about a hundred years ago, right after penicillin was invented." She laughed, and so did I.

I remembered my first day at the hospital in Dallas, when I was just out of training, and was told there were two sick patients in the emergency room waiting on me. On my second day in Dallas, I was sued because I had the misfortune to be walking past the cardiac catheterization lab as a patient was having a cardiac arrest. I was called in to help, the patient ultimately died, and the ensuing lawsuit named me as a defendant. *That* was my orientation; there was no touchy-feely get-to-know-you session. This whole concept was quite new.

We spent time reviewing the vision and mission of the hospital, grandiose statements put together by a committee that no doubt spent countless hours with marketing folks, wordsmithing the language until the statements were indistinguishable from similar statements by any other hospital.

Looking at the hospital mission and vision statements projected up on a huge screen in that conference room reminded me of the T-shirts we wore as residents. "Parkland Hospital: Greet 'Em, Treat 'Em, and Street 'Em." I guess that wouldn't get out of the vision and mission committees in any hospital today, but it, indelicately, described what we were there to do. Thinking back, it was a reminder of just how much the hospital culture had changed. Egomaniacs treating patients like widgets on an assembly line were no longer tolerated. Nor should they be.

This was going to be interesting.

The session began with some opening comments and then a "get to know each other" exercise that took me a bit by surprise. The leader asked us to share family photos with one another. As we passed our phones around, looking at each other's photos—my teenage daughters, their babies in onesies—we complimented each other's beautiful families.

I wondered, *What do the people at this table think, that I came to medicine late, after doing something else? Maybe a radiology technician? And that's why I'm at the orientation?*

The rest of the morning was spent on a variety of topics, including the patient experience, communication, and teamwork. There was also time spent on something for which I didn't even know there was a name: Distracted Healthcare. *Was there any other kind of healthcare except distracted healthcare?* The whole job is full of interruptions and distractions of all kinds, from pages from the nurses and calls on our cell phones from referring physicians to buzzers and alarms in the ICU. But the discussion centered around a new way for physicians to get themselves in trouble: malpractice, presumably because mistakes were made while a physician was on their phone. Whether the doctor was doing something related to their job (or buying something on Amazon) was unclear, but the technology poses a whole new challenge in the already challenging environment of practicing medicine in a hospital.

All these areas are certainly important, but there were also surprising new areas of discussion among healthcare providers. I had been out of a hospital only two years, but it could have been twenty. The faces of the other people had changed (younger), the city had changed (hotter), and the language in the hospital had changed. Instead of just giving us our badges and telling us to get out there and get to work, we were now instructed on how to interact with our colleagues, compassionately care for our patients—that is, tell them what's wrong with them and what we plan to do about it, but moreover actually listen to them, and them ask if they understood what we were telling them.

The last presentation got my attention: a discussion of physician burnout by someone with the title of chief wellness officer, a title I found so forward-thinking, so hopeful. Ochsner, like more and more hospitals, had a department devoted to considering how the people who worked at the hospital were coping and planning strategies to deal with times when providers weren't doing so well. Progress.

Standing outside the door to the clinic room where I would see my first patient in two years, I thought, *Piece of cake. This is the part you do well. Talking with patients and their families alone.* I took a deep breath and swung open the door.

Waiting inside was a fifty-five-year-old black woman named Deborah who had emphysema. I greeted her, introducing myself as I took one of her hands in both of mine. With her were two kids who appeared to be in their twenties, a daughter wearing a T-shirt that said "Love Trumps Hate" and a son dressed in a black tracksuit.

This beautiful woman with sad eyes was my age but was facing very different results from her roll of the dice. She wanted to be able to volunteer at her church, cook lunch for the Sunday parishioners, and sing in her church choir. There are no words to describe how it felt that day to hear this sweet woman's simple aspirations if she were to get a transplant and survive. *What a blessing to be back in this room*, I thought. For more than two years I had been away from these conversations, these unique human experiences, and the connectedness they enabled me to feel.

I was going through some of the more mundane mechanics of getting her on the waiting list—imploring her to remain abstinent from cigarette smoking for six months, a follow-up CT chest scan, enrollment in physical therapy—when a white middle-aged man came into the room without knocking.

He and the patient embraced. *Who is this guy? Husband? Friend?*

It turned out, Deborah had had three children. The third, a son, had died a year earlier. And this man had her deceased son's heart in his chest. The patient for whom I was trying to get a new set of lungs already had experience with the donor process and transplantation. She consented for her son's heart to go a stranger, to whom she would clearly be bonded to forever.

I watch them hold an embrace, eyes closed, tears flowing. Her tragedy, his gain, his gratitude, her love. *I bear witness to this grace, this moment.*

I told her that I understood the hurt, that I hurt for her. I reached out for the patient's hand and took hold of it, while her son's heart recipient still held the other.

These are the times.

I find myself in the clinic room with these people, whom I do not know, but I am now better than when I entered the room. It's worth it: the hospital rules, the egos, the burden of the responsibility. In these moments, as an observer of the best in people, I get what I need, what we all need. The education of a lifetime.

An education in how inherently good people can be. When they suffer, when they give help, when they need help. Maybe—just maybe—some of this will rub off on me, some of this good will overshadow all that is bad in others, in me. That's why I wanted to do this so badly, and that's why I had come back. So I have the opportunity to experience something special. So I can have the opportunity to be better.

I see that now.

I couldn't see it as well when I was moving through the hospital so fast, through life so fast. Being back in the hospital, even in a limited way, was a step. I find I'm hopeful for the first time in years. This time, I will savor the experience and be mindful of its impact on the people I treat, on the people I work with, on my family—and on me.

And as I sat there in that clinic room—with people I had met just a few minutes before—I felt connected. I felt good. I felt I had come back to myself.

Only one word came to mind.

Slowly.

Slowly.

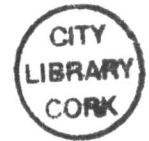

Acknowledgments

Writing a book can be lonely at times. There was no team of people with me every day like I had rounding in the hospital, no one with whom to exchange barbs and banter, no one with whom to celebrate when good sentences, paragraphs, then pages happened—and no one with whom to commiserate when the blank page overwhelmed.

But I never felt alone writing this book because of the many people who helped me along the way. I'd like to thank some of them.

First, to Claire Wachtel, who provided editorial direction and taught me far more about writing than anyone I've ever encountered and who frequently reminded me that writing is hard, but numbering my pages shouldn't be. She is right on both counts.

To my agent, Mel Parker of Mel Parker Books, who from the beginning, believed in the work of this first-time author. That meant everything to me.

To the professionals at Post Hill Press, especially Debby Englander and Heather King, who guided me through the publishing maze with skill and patience.

To Moshe Schulman, of Schulman PR, who believed in my project and worked tirelessly to get the word out about the book.

To the early readers of my "vomit drafts"—especially Judy Weill and Leslie Ehret, who were quick to point out where I got something wrong…as only older sisters reliably can. And to Gene Lafitte, who read each word as it came out, chapter by chapter, and always had a unique perspective about how to make the book better and an even more unique way of telling me how to do so. I am sorry he can't see the final product.

To Brooke Warner, who taught me the fundamentals of memoir writing and had the fortitude to read the early drafts when my writing left a great deal to be desired. To the extent the writing has improved at all, Brooke had a hand in that. If the writing still isn't up to par, she should be held blameless.

To Mallory Smith, who did two things that I won't forget: one, she helped with early edits; and two, more importantly, gave me the privilege of being one of her doctors.

To Karl Weber, who sat in the dining room with me and taught me about story shape—an underrated concept that, before meeting Karl, had eluded me.

To Dani Shapiro, who for many years through her own writing, has shown me that writing a memoir can lead to understanding and healing. To have her work with me on my writing is a dream come true. I'll never forget the central theme of her teaching: what we write about chooses us and announces itself—it scares us and needs to be written.

To Terence Blanchard, who provided the soundtrack while I wrote. My "art" will never approach his art, but every day as I wrote, he gave me something to which to aspire. You can score my movie—or my life, for that matter—any time, TB.

To my colleagues at Weill Consulting Group—Pete Tafaro, Shelley Hewitt, Trish Magee, Meredith Waldron, and Jackie Weill—who gave me the space, time, and quiet(!) to write.

And, finally, to my patients: Your stories and your courage get me out of bed each day, trying to do the best I can. Any sacrifice I've made to take care of you pales in comparison to the sacrifices you make every day just to stay alive. You gave me the education of a lifetime for which I'll always be grateful.